T0254426

Law and Ethics in Complementary Medicine

Comprehensive, practical and reflective of the current Australian and New Zealand legislative framework and regulations, this unique textbook addresses legal and ethical issues across a broad range of traditional and complementary practices. The sixth edition of Michael Weir's classic textbook:

- explores legal and ethical issues in clinical relationships, and the role of codes of ethics;
- provides practical guidelines for setting up and running a professional practice;
- systematically outlines the various aspects of the law which impact on clinical practice, including legal obligations to clients, consumer legislation, complaints processes, and professional boundaries;
- explains how to navigate professional indemnity insurance;
- outlines the steps you need to take in setting up a professional practice from establishing a business name to dealing with employees;
- discusses and provides examples of how to deal with tricky ethical issues in daily practice.

This edition includes updated legislation, a review of relevant case law, recent developments in the Unregistered Practitioners' Code of Conduct and evidence about misconduct and regulatory action, and more in-depth discussion of ethical concepts. This is an essential read for students and practitioners of complementary medicine.

Michael Weir is Professor in the Faculty of Law at Bond University, Australia.

Law and Ethics in Complementary Medicine

A Handbook for Practitioners
in Australia and New Zealand

6th edition

Michael Weir

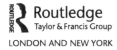

LONDON AND NEW YORK

Cover image: John Lauriat

Sixth edition published 2023
by Routledge
4 Park Square, Milton Park, Abingdon, Oxon, OX14 4RN

and by Routledge
605 Third Avenue, New York, NY 10158

Routledge is an imprint of the Taylor & Francis Group, an informa business

First edition published by Routledge 2000
Fifth edition published by Routledge 2020

British Library Cataloguing-in-Publication Data
A catalogue record for this book is available from the British Library

Library of Congress Cataloging-in-Publication Data
Names: Weir, Michael, 1957- author.
Title: Law and ethics in complementary medicine : a handbook for practitioners in Australia and New Zealand / Michael Weir.
Description: Sixth edition. | Abingdon, Oxon ; New York, NY : Routledge, 2022. | Includes bibliographical references and index.
Identifiers: LCCN 2022014275 (print) | LCCN 2022014276 (ebook) | ISBN 9781032050881 (hbk) | ISBN 9781032050867 (pbk) | ISBN 9781003195931 (ebk)
Subjects: LCSH: Medical laws and legislation--Australia. | Alternative medicine--Law and legislation--Australia. | Alternative medicine--Moral and ethical aspects--Australia. | Medical ethics--Australia. | Medical laws and legislation--New Zealand. | Alternative medicine--Law and legislation--New Zealand. | Alternative medicine--Moral and ethical aspects--New Zealand. | Medical ethics--New Zealand.
Classification: LCC KU1520 .W45 2022 (print) | LCC KU1520 (ebook) | DDC 344.9404/1--dc23/eng/20220801
LC record available at https://lccn.loc.gov/2022014275
LC ebook record available at https://lccn.loc.gov/2022014276

ISBN: 978-1-032-05088-1 (hbk)
ISBN: 978-1-032-05086-7 (pbk)
ISBN: 978-1-003-19593-1 (ebk)

DOI: 10.4324/9781003195931

Typeset in Times New Roman
by KnowledgeWorks Global Ltd.

To my darling Elana and Matthew.

Contents

Preface

This 6th edition provides an update of the development of legal and ethical matters for complementary medicine in both Australia and New Zealand. The primary issues that have been added or developed includes:

- Ethical concepts relevant to practice of complementary medicine
- Privacy and the application of the recently promulgated *Guide to health privacy*
- Updates in AHPRA requirements, Codes and Guidelines
- Updated details about the development of the National Code of Conduct for Unregistered Practitioners
- New information and developments under the *Therapeutic Goods Act*
- Incorporation of new relevant case law
- Updates of significant issues for specific modalities including Chiropractic, Chinese medicine and Therapeutic Massage.

In this edition the chapter on 'The Legal Process' has been moved from Chapter 8 to Chapter 2, based upon requests from readers. It is important to understand that the continuing development of legal and ethical issues and burgeoning complexity of that area suggests the need to seek legal, accounting or other expert advice in making decisions.

This work deals with matters relevant to Australia and New Zealand and it is appropriate to acknowledge in this preface that the Māori name for New Zealand is Aotearoa. I acknowledge and thank the staff of Routledge for their assistance in the preparation of this edition. As far as possible the law is to 30 January 2022.

1   Introduction

Successful professional practice requires technical, business and personal skills, as well as an ability to deal with a rapidly changing profession, society and economy. An understanding of where your modality fits into the health sector can help with these challenging requirements. This chapter offers a short overview of what complementary medicine is and how it is regulated.

The Ten Commandments of Professional Practice at the end of this chapter summarise the most important themes of the book. By understanding and integrating these principles into day-to-day practice, a health practitioner will not only earn the respect of clients and colleagues, but will create a more successful and enjoyable practice.

BOX 1.1

Action plan

- Investigate and appreciate your role and that of your modality in complementary medicine.
- Read and understand the Ten Commandments of Professional Practice.
- Understand that you are a professional.

What is complementary medicine?

Looking at different ways to approach the healing process can clarify how a practitioner fits into the healthcare industry and how he or she relates to other health professionals.

Terminology

Complementary medicine is that part of the health sector that relies primarily upon holistic, homoeopathic, traditional or natural therapies rather than an allopathic approach to medicine, which characterises Western or orthodox medicine. The World Health Organization provides a definition:

> The terms 'complementary medicine' or 'alternative medicine' refer to a broad set of healthcare practices that are not part of that country's own tradition or

DOI: 10.4324/9781003195931-1

conventional medicine and are not fully integrated into the dominant health-care system. They are used interchangeably with traditional medicine in some countries.[1]

This book is useful for all complementary medicine practitioners but will deal specifically with:

- acupuncture
- chiropractic
- herbal medicine
- homoeopathy
- holistic counselling
- naturopathy
- osteopathy
- therapeutic massage and myotherapy
- traditional Chinese medicine
- yoga

In this book, we focus on a broad spectrum of modalities, and it is necessary to refer to all of them. It can be difficult to find a term that adequately covers all modalities, techniques or systems because they often exhibit contrasting philosophies and approaches, so in this book the term 'complementary medicine' is applied. This appears to provoke the least philosophical objection for the majority of modalities. Some may bridle at the suggestion that their modality is complementary to anything. Some will perceive their modality as all-encompassing and complete in itself. Others will be relaxed with this terminology. The focus of the book is not upon the provision of complementary medicine by orthodox medicine practitioners, though most of the book will provide insights for these integrative practitioners.

The term 'natural therapies' is accepted by some and understood by many laypeople, but some therapies are not particularly natural. The term 'alternative medicine' was considered, but this may differentiate it unnecessarily from orthodox medicine. Many modalities have grown out of traditional medicine, so some reference to traditional medicine may be suggested. These modalities may have little in common with newer modalities. The terms 'complementary and alternative medicine' (CAM) or 'traditional, complementary and integrative medicine' (TCIM) are in common parlance, but they are somewhat clumsy to use in the title and throughout the book.

The term 'complementary medicine' therefore has been chosen as a useful and inclusive description of the modalities discussed in this book. The use of this term is not intended to exclude or sideline any particular approach or philosophy in order to limit the role played by complementary medicine or its potential as an alternative therapy in the health sector.

Approaches to healing

The various philosophies and approaches to treatment used in complementary medicine are hard to categorise, but a helpful starting point is to compare allopathic and homoeopathic approaches. Orthodox medicine is based on an allopathic approach to healing. The practitioner introduces into the body substances (such as pharmaceutical products) designed to counteract the effect of symptoms of disease or injury, and may use invasive procedures such as surgery. An allopath generally regards the human body as a machine made of many parts, and the doctor as an expert who 'fixes the body'. An allopath will seek to fix the diseased or injured part without necessarily focusing on the body as a whole.

In contrast, a homoeopath's aim is not to counteract disease but rather to stimulate a healing response. Homoeopathy is based on the principles of similars—that is, a homoeopath introduces into the body tiny amounts of a substance to produce an effect similar to the disease symptoms, aiming to stimulate the healing response. Other modalities share a 'holistic' approach to healing that perceives the body as a whole system. Rather than focusing on the disease state itself, the practitioner assesses how imbalance in the body may be contributing to ill-health. The task of the practitioner is to restore balance and equilibrium to the body.

Complementary medicine practitioners may on occasion use a symptomatic approach influenced by allopathy. A practitioner may apply different modalities such as kinesiology, acupuncture, therapeutic massage and naturopathy, each of them different in approach but directed towards the goal of bringing harmony and balance to the body. The less authoritarian therapeutic relationship preferred by complementary medicine practitioners, involving more a health partnership between practitioner and client, is reflected in the use of the term 'client' in this book, as distinct from the term 'patient'.

Categories of complementary medicine

One way to understand how the various modalities of complementary medicine relate to each other is to divide them into four general types:[2]

1 *Complete systems of healing* such as acupuncture, traditional Chinese medicine, herbal medicine, osteopathy, chiropractic, homoeopathy and naturopathy. These disciplines seek to provide complete explanations of the cause of disease, though most practitioners do acknowledge the boundaries of the discipline and the role to be played by orthodox medicine. This book will explore in some detail where these boundaries should be drawn for the benefit of clients and practitioners.
2 *Diagnostic methods* such as iridology, kinesiology and aura analysis. Some practitioners may rely heavily on these methods, while practitioners of complete healing systems will often use them to detect disease, abnormality or imbalance. For example, a chiropractor may use kinesiology to help diagnose a misaligned spine or a naturopath may use iridology to diagnose imbalances in the body or organs.
3 *Therapeutic modalities* such as musculoskeletal therapy, therapeutic massage and myotherapy, reflexology, aromatherapy, spiritual healing, holistic counselling and shiatsu. These modalities emphasise therapeutic effect rather than diagnosis. For example, a practitioner of therapeutic massage may aim to heighten the recipient's sense of well-being rather than to alleviate any particular diagnosed illness, though that might be the result of the treatment. In some cases, such as in therapeutic massage and musculoskeletal therapy, the focus of the treatment may be on dealing with a specific injury or pain.
4 *Self-help measures* such as relaxation, yoga, qi dong, tai chi, meditation, guided visualisation or fasting.

Regulation of health professionals

Regulation of health professionals defines appropriate roles for complementary medicine practitioners in the healthcare sector.

Models of regulation

Regulators tend to focus on the role of complete systems of healing because they provide a greater risk of harm. For example, traditional Chinese medicine involves the ingestion of herbs, acupuncture involves the piercing of the skin and chiropractic involves manipulation of the spine, which may involve an element of risk.

Orthodox medicine has had a profound effect on the regulation of complementary medicine. In the United Kingdom, orthodox medicine rose to pre-eminence over other traditional forms of healing during the course of the fifteenth century. The process culminated in the *Medical Act 1858* (UK), which gave state endorsement and protection for orthodox medicine.[3] This history has to a great extent been mirrored in Australia.

Medical practitioners and other allied health professionals—such as physiotherapists, optometrists and podiatrists—work within subsets of medical practice as primary health practitioners, and are recognised by state legislation based upon a national health practitioner legislative scheme discussed in Chapter 3.

Osteopaths, chiropractors and practitioners of traditional Chinese medicine, acupuncturists and Chinese medicine dispensers are also registered health practitioners in Australia. All other complementary medicine practitioners are unregistered health professionals. The unregistered complementary medicine practitioners—for example, therapeutic massage therapists, homoeopaths, naturopaths and herbal medicine practitioners—need to be aware of a few statutorily defined restricted acts that only specified registered health practitioners can perform. All health professions are also regulated by other significant common law and statutory limitations. The regulatory structure that applies to complementary medicine practitioners will be discussed further in Chapter 3.

The regulation of the health sector in Australia follows one of three models: statutory regulation, voluntary self-regulation or negative licensing.

STATUTORY REGULATION

Statutory regulation of health professions in Australia is established by state and territory legislation, based upon an agreement reached between the states for a 'National Law' to regulate registered health practitioners through a national model of regulation. The National Law creates separate national registration boards for each registered health profession. There are some differences between each state statute and the National Law, especially in relation to discipline procedures. Each national registration board maintains a register of health professionals who must comply with prescribed educational, health and personal character standards. The National Law includes protection of title provisions and a small number of restricted acts that may be performed only by specified registered health practitioners.

Protection of title provisions permits only registrants to use particular titles, such as 'physiotherapist' or 'podiatrist', that are relevant to the registered profession. The statute penalises the use of those titles by non-registrants. An example of a restricted act under the National Law is high-velocity cervical spine manipulation, which can only be performed by osteopaths, chiropractors, medical doctors and physiotherapists.

Statutory regulation applies to a large number of health professions, including medical practice, physiotherapy, podiatry, chiropractic and osteopathy. It provides the legal basis to enforce standards of practice through penalties such as deregistration or suspension, backed up in appropriate cases by criminal sanctions.[4] Statutory regulation allows the application and enforcement of standardised qualifications, adherence to professional ethics and the requirement for registrants to involve themselves in continuing professional education.[5]

VOLUNTARY SELF-REGULATION

This model envisages each modality policing its own professional ethical standards, normally through a professional association code of ethics or code of practice. The specific provisions contained in these codes attempt to define, promote and enforce ethical practice. The most serious disciplinary measure (suspension or exclusion from the association) does not prevent a practitioner from continuing to practise without the advantages of membership. Currently, most complementary medicine practitioners are regulated in this way. Some unregistered complementary medicine practitioners are not members of a professional association.

Even if practitioners are subject to specific statutory regulation and/or voluntary self-regulation, all practitioners are also subject to criminal and civil law sanctions. This includes being subject to an action in negligence or being charged with a criminal offence. Practitioners may also be subject to consumer legislation such as the various state *Fair Trading Acts* and the Commonwealth *Competition and Consumer Act 2010*.

NEGATIVE LICENSING

A decision was made by the Council of Australian Governments Health Council (now known as the Health Council) in 2015 to apply a National Code of Conduct for Health Care Workers as discussed later in this book.[6] To date New South Wales, Queensland, South Australia and Victoria have introduced a statutory Code of Conduct for Unregistered Health Practitioners which set out required performance standards for those subject to the Code. Tasmania has passed legislation for a Code of Conduct but as not yet enacted that initiative. A significant aspect of these codes and associated legislation is that it provides the capacity to grant prohibition orders against practitioners who breach the terms of the Code of Conduct. This provides greater capacity to regulate unregistered health practitioners without the costs of formal registration. This form of regulation, called 'negative licensing', involves allowing persons to provide health services with limited regulation, but regulatory action may arise if a breach of a code of conduct occurs or some illegal act is committed, triggering action under the enforcement powers granted by relevant legislation.

Ten Commandments of professional practice

The Ten Commandments of Professional Practice provide the stepping stones for reaching the goal of competent and ethical professional practice. These commandments summarise the main themes of this book, describing actions that promote better, more professional and more successful practice.

Table 1.1 Ten commandments of professional practice

Commandment	Relevant chapter of the book
1. I shall practise in a competent, caring and responsible manner.	Chapters 3 and 5
2. I shall keep up to date with developments in clinical techniques and professional and social issues.	Chapters 3, 5, 7
3. I shall practise within the scope of my expertise and understand and respect my limitations.	Chapter 4
4. I shall practise from premises and use substances that are safe, legally compliant and conducive to the healing process.	Chapters 6, 8 and pages 142–154 and 203–219
5. I shall practise in accordance with professional ethical principles and the ethical precepts of my profession.	Chapter 3
6. I shall compile, secure and maintain thorough and legible client records.	Chapter 3 pages 58–61
7. I shall maintain professional indemnity insurance for the protection of my client and myself.	Chapter 8 and pages 225–230
8. I shall respect the confidence of the therapeutic relationship to promote trust and confidence in my profession and myself.	Chapter 3 pages 49–57
9. I shall provide accurate and sufficient information and advice to my client to allow proper decision-making and consent to treatment.	Chapter 5 pages 122–131
10. I shall place my client's interests above my own.	Chapter 3

Notes

1 https://www.who.int/health-topics/traditional-complementary-and-integrative-medicine (accessed 10 July 2021).
2 J. Stone & J. Matthews, *Complementary Medicine and the Law*, Oxford University Press, Oxford, 1996, pp. 88–9.
3 Ibid., Ch. 1; M. Weir, *Alternative Medicine: A New Regulatory Model*, Australian Scholarly Press, Melbourne, 2005, pp. 48–100.
4 Stone & Matthews, *Complementary Medicine and the Law*, p. 157.
5 Ibid., p. 158.
6 https://www.coaghealthcouncil.gov.au/NationalCodeOfConductForHealthCareWorkers (accessed 10 July 2021).

2   The legal process

Complementary medicine practitioners perform their professional tasks in a legal environment. An appreciation of the basic features of the legal structure is helpful for understanding obligations and entitlements. Most of the relevant law is found in statutes or regulations passed by federal or state parliaments, or in the common law laid down in legal precedent by judges.

Practitioners may act as a witness, either as an expert in a claim against another practitioner or as a witness in a claim for or against themselves. A practitioner with some basic understanding of the role of a witness is better equipped to deal with the potentially bewildering nature of courtroom procedure.

BOX 2.1

Action plan

- Understand the basic structure of our legal system.
- Understand what happens in court if you are a witness.
- Understand your role as an expert witness.

Sources of law in Australia

Our law derives from:

- statutes (the laws passed by parliament)
- delegated legislation (includes regulations made by governments and local authority by-laws)
- the common law (law made by judges in court decisions)
- the rules of equity (rules based on concepts of fairness and equity that evolved to overcome some of the harshness of the common law), and
- international law.

Much of our law derives originally from our legal and historical connection to England and English common law.

DOI: 10.4324/9781003195931-2

Common law: Doctrine of precedent

The common law develops over time based on judges' decisions. If a court determines a matter based on a principle of law applicable to a particular set of facts, a lower court within the same judicial system is obliged to apply that precedent to subsequent cases. The process is an application of 'the doctrine of precedent'. Sometimes a judge might decide to apply a different principle of law if he or she determines that the facts are not the same as or comparable to those dealt with in the previous decision. In that situation, a judge is said to 'distinguish' this case.

Statute

Statute is legislation passed by one of the parliaments in Australia—that is, the parliaments of the Commonwealth, the six states and the two territories. These statutes may bring new law into existence, repeal current statutes or override common law principles no longer appropriate to society. Some statutes provide a comprehensive treatment of one area of the law so as to exclude the common law entirely. This type of statute is called a code. An example is the Criminal Code of Queensland, which provides a comprehensive statement of the principles of Queensland's criminal law. The very extensive use of statutes in most areas of human activity has meant that judges are becoming increasingly concerned with the interpretation of statutes and determining the extent of their impact on a broad range of activities.

Constitutional issues: Impact on law-making

Australia has a federal system of government with a central Commonwealth government, six states and two territories. The Commonwealth government has a written constitution set out in the *Constitution of the Commonwealth of Australia Act 1900*. Each of the states has its own written constitution. The constitutions of the Commonwealth and state governments define the scope of the powers of these parliaments to pass laws.

Commonwealth Constitution

A feature of the Commonwealth Constitution is that it contains a list of powers, which provides the basis upon which the Commonwealth can validly pass legislation. These include matters such as defence or foreign affairs. These powers are exercisable by the Commonwealth as well as by the states. This can and does lead to conflict with state laws. Section 109 of the Constitution states that a Commonwealth statute will prevail if there is inconsistency with state legislation. Some powers of the Commonwealth are exclusive to the Commonwealth—for example, the power to impose customs and excise duties.

State constitutions

The constitutions of the states don't specify a list of powers; rather, they generally indicate that the states have broad powers to make laws for 'the peace, welfare and good government of the State'. The limits of the state's power are found when inconsistency with Commonwealth laws occurs or in relation to powers exclusive to the

Commonwealth. For example, a state could seek to legislate in relation to a matter relevant to defence, but this is likely to be inconsistent with Commonwealth legislation.

New Zealand

As there are no states in New Zealand, the complexity of constitutional issues between the Commonwealth and state powers does not arise. The national government derives its ability to pass laws based upon the terms of the *Constitution Act 1986*.

Impact of constitutional limitations

The limits on Commonwealth powers affect the ability of the Commonwealth to legislate for many activities. For example, the Commonwealth *Therapeutic Goods Act 1989* has a limited scope because the Commonwealth can only legislate in relation to trade and commerce across state or national borders or by corporations. Transactions on intrastate matters by individuals are constitutionally outside the purview of this legislation. This is why the full impact of that legislation is only felt when states enact complementary legislation that deals with intrastate transactions. This has now occurred in Victoria, Tasmania, South Australia, Queensland and New South Wales (refer to page 144).

In some cases, to provide national legislative regimes where the Commonwealth lacks constitutional power, the Commonwealth and the states have entered into an intergovernmental agreement in which all the states agree to pass the same or very similar legislation. This occurred in regard to the National Law discussed in Chapter 4 in relation to national health profession legislation.

Types of law

There are a number of different classifications or types of law.

Public/private law

One very broad classification relates to public and private law:

- Public law relates to matters between government and government, and between people and government. Examples are constitutional law, administrative law and criminal law.
- Private law relates to matters relevant to individuals and organisations.

Some private law areas could briefly be described as:

- *contract law*: the law relating to binding civil obligations between parties and the means by which those contracts can be varied, terminated and enforced
- *torts law*: the law of civil wrongs, encompassing the obligation to avoid negligent or careless conduct that might injure one's neighbour, the law in relation to trespass to land and goods, and defamation
- *property law*: the law relating to the enforcement of rights in land and personal property, and

- *succession law*: the law relative to succession of property on the death of a person, based on the terms of a will or the rules of intestacy. The rules of intestacy are the statutory rules that apply when a person dies without a valid will.

Civil/criminal law

Another way to classify law is to distinguish between civil and criminal law:

- *civil law* involves an individual, organisation or government seeking a private remedy, whether it is by way of damages or by enforcement of a contract.
- *criminal law* relates to offences committed against the state, although it will often relate to an act such as theft that affects an individual or company. The state, through the instrument of the police and prosecutors of the state or Commonwealth government, enforces the relevant statute or common law that has been breached.

Parties to a dispute

In civil proceedings, the party who commences the action is 'the plaintiff' and the person sued by the plaintiff is 'the defendant'. If either party appeals against the decision of a court to a higher court, they are called 'the appellant' and the party resisting the appeal is 'the respondent'. In criminal matters, the state is deemed 'the prosecution' and the party charged is 'the accused'.

Standard of proof

An important distinction between civil and criminal proceedings is the standard of proof that applies. In the civil jurisdiction, the plaintiff needs to prove their case 'on the balance of probabilities'. The standard of proof for the prosecution in the criminal jurisdiction is the much higher standard of proof 'beyond reasonable doubt'.

Court system

In Australia, there are two court systems that dispense justice: the state courts that derive their jurisdiction from state laws and the federal courts that derive their jurisdiction from the Commonwealth government. The apex of both systems is the High Court of Australia.

State judicial hierarchy

On most matters, an appeal to the High Court requires the High Court to give leave to appeal—that is, an appeal is not as of right. The High Court deals with all matters that relate to the interpretation of the Commonwealth Constitution. The High Court consists of seven justices. In significant cases, all seven justices will hear the appeal. The state judicial hierarchy comprises the following:

1 The apex is the High Court.
2 Each state has a Court of Appeal or Full Court and a Court of Criminal Appeal. This court, normally constituting three justices, hears appeals against decisions of lower courts.

3 Each state has a Supreme Court, normally with a single judge who will hear significant civil and criminal matters.
4 Each state has a District Court or County Court that hears a wide range of lower
  value civil matters and criminal matters.
5 Each state has a Local or Magistrates Court that hears petty criminal law matters
  or smaller civil claims. The court will also hear committal proceedings for serious
  criminal matters such as murder to determine whether the accused has a case to
  answer before the matter proceeds to a higher court for hearing. There may be an
  appeal to the District or Supreme Court from a decision of a magistrate.

Federal judicial hierarchy

1 High Court of Australia. The High Court hears appeals from decisions of Federal
  Courts and tribunals.
2 a Full Court of the Federal Court. This court hears appeals from the Federal
       Court and is normally constituted by three Federal Court judges.

   b Full Court of the Family Court. This court hears appeals from the Family
       Court and Federal Magistrates Court.

3 a Federal Court of Australia.

   b Family Court of Australia.

4 Federal Magistrates Court. This court deals with matters that arise on
  Commonwealth statutes, including the *Family Law Act 1975* (Cth).

New Zealand court system

The New Zealand court system does not have the same complexity (caused by the
different state and federal courts) that applies in Australia.

1 The Supreme Court is at the apex of the court system in New Zealand and is the
  final court of appeal in New Zealand.
2 The Court of Appeal hears appeals from the High Court and appeals from more
  serious criminal matters in the District Court.
3 The High Court deals with matters at first instance or appeals from lower courts
  on civil and criminal matters.
4 The District Court deals with minor criminal and civil matters and is probably
  equivalent to the Magistrates Court in Australia.
5 The Maori Land Court, Coroners Court, Employment Court, Environment
  Court, Youth Court and Family Court complete the system.

Acting as a witness

A practitioner may be required to provide evidence to a court or tribunal, either as
part of a claim made against them in their professional capacity or as an expert witness. This section will outline the major issues relevant to fulfilling the role of witness
or expert witness. Our court system has a preference for evidence provided by the oral
testimony of witnesses although, in some proceedings, evidence may be adduced by

written affidavit. A person is considered more likely to be truthful if they testify in person under oath or affirmation.

What happens in court?

A witness will first be called to the witness stand and asked to swear or affirm that the evidence they give will be 'the truth the whole truth and nothing but the truth'. The witness will then be subject to interrogation, covering:

* *evidence in chief* (the provision of evidence by the party calling that witness)
* *cross-examination* (questioning by the opposing party), and
* *re-examination* (further questions by the party calling the witness).

The witness provides evidence by answering the questions put to him or her.[1]

Evidence in chief

During evidence in chief, counsel for the witness will ask questions of the witness and elicit replies. Counsel is not entitled to ask leading questions—that is, questions suggesting the answer. An example of a leading question might be: 'On 10 October 2020 in the accused's office did the accused indecently assault you while providing a massage?' This information should be elicited by questions such as: 'Where were you on 10 October 2020?' 'What services did the accused contract to perform for you?' 'What happened during this massage?' Leading questions are not permitted as they may put words in the mouth of the witness.

   The general rule is that witnesses are obliged to give evidence based on their perceptions, and are not entitled to give opinions or inferences from data or observable circumstances.[2] Thus it would not be appropriate for a witness to simply provide evidence that a person was negligent; rather, the witness should describe the precautions the defendant did or did not observe. This is a difficult rule to apply absolutely, as it is inevitable that some form of inference is required when making any observation. The rule against opinion evidence does not apply where the opinion is based on what the person saw, heard or perceived, and evidence of the opinion is necessary to obtain an adequate account or understanding of the person's perception.[3] Examples of opinions that might be permitted are:

* identification of handwriting, persons or things
* the emotional state of a person
* the condition of things (e.g. they looked old, new or used), and
* the condition of a person (e.g. they looked ill).

Cross-examination

In cross-examination, the intention of the opposing counsel is to damage the credibility of the witness and to elicit from the witness facts or information that might be favourable to the case of their client. In cross-examination, leading questions can be asked, assuming that they are not unfair or likely to evince misleading answers. The frustration for a witness in cross-examination is that a skilled advocate with carefully crafted questions can evince answers to create a negative inference.

Re-examination

Re-examination provides an opportunity for a witness to qualify evidence or to deal with ambiguities that may have arisen on cross-examination. Re-examination is limited to matters that have arisen out of cross-examination. Leading questions are not permitted.

Expert witnesses

An exception to the rule prohibiting opinion evidence relates to expert evidence. Where the matter at issue calls for specialist training and/or experience, opinion evidence of an expert witness is admissible:[4] 'The opinion of the expert is a substitute for speculation by the court in an area where the court is unskilled.'[5]

A senior complementary medicine practitioner may become involved as an expert in circumstances of:[6]

- litigation relating to workers' compensation and motor vehicle accidents
- criminal charges relating to professional misconduct, and
- professional negligence litigation.

Workers' compensation and motor vehicle accidents

In Commonwealth legislation and in all states, there is provision for workers' compensation to be paid in relation to chiropractic and often osteopathic care and in some cases for therapeutic massage.[7] The Commonwealth, Victoria and South Australia allow chiropractors to certify time off for employees. In relation to transport accident legislation, there is partial or full provision for coverage for chiropractic care in New South Wales, Victoria, South Australia, Western Australia, Tasmania and the Australian Capital Territory.[8]

Increasingly, complementary medicine practitioners are becoming integrated and accepted into medical rehabilitation and compensation schemes. In one Accident Compensation Tribunal decision, the expert evidence of a chiropractor as to the injury sustained by an employee in the course of his employment was preferred to the evidence of an orthopaedic specialist. The orthopaedic specialist had argued that the injury was inherent and not caused by his employment. The chiropractor was deemed to be providing appropriate treatment for the injured party.[9]

The use of expert reports regarding the medical condition of a plaintiff seeking recovery of personal injuries for an accident will likely be confined to medical doctors and, on occasion, chiropractors. In jury cases, where the plaintiff has been treated by a chiropractor after an accident, it is desirable to get an expert report from such a practitioner. The chiropractor is competent to testify as a medical witness or an expert concerning matters within the scope of his or her profession and practice as a chiropractor. Within this field, a chiropractor may have qualifications to interpret x-rays and express his or her opinion as to the probable cause of the patient's injury and its permanency.[10]

Criminal cases involving professional misconduct

On occasion, it is necessary for a practitioner to provide evidence to a court as to the nature of a technique and normal professional procedures. In *MJM v R*,[11] an officer of a professional massage association was called as an expert witness to give evidence regarding what was acceptable professional practice for a polarity massage therapist charged with rape.

One ground of the appeal against the conviction was that the inclusion of this evidence was prejudicial to the accused. It is significant that the court accepted that the witness was an expert in the area, although she did not practise in the speciality of polarity massage therapy. This evidence was adduced to determine what might be appropriate procedures to avoid unnecessary exposure or contact with genital areas. The court held that the use of the evidence of that expert was appropriate in the circumstances.

Professional negligence litigation

The important issue in professional negligence litigation is whether the practitioner has satisfied the appropriate duty of care. To determine this issue, a court will normally require evidence of the standard procedures for a professional in the circumstances in which the practitioner found him or herself. The civil liability legislation that applies to the negligence liability of 'professionals' requires a court to consider peer professional opinion to determine whether negligence has occurred (refer to pages 101–102, 104, 115, 123). If the matter relates to a practitioner not considered to be a 'professional' the common law test relates to the standard of a reasonably competent member of that group. For these reasons, reference to evidence of an accomplished member of the profession will often be required.

Choosing an expert witness

Before expert evidence is admitted, there are a number of issues to be determined:

- *Does the jury or judge need assistance?* If a court can reach its own conclusions, then expert evidence may not be necessary. For example, if the matter at issue in the proceeding was the tendency for acupuncture to induce light-headedness, this would probably require expert evidence. If the issue was whether water left on a polished floor of a clinic could make the floor slippery, a court may consider that this does not require expert evidence. Expert evidence might still be of assistance in determining the normal precautions taken to deal with slippery floors.
- *Is there a recognised area of expertise?* An expert can only give evidence as an expert if they have knowledge in an area that is a recognised area of expertise. The court will ask 'whether the subject matter of the opinion forms part of a body of knowledge or experience that is sufficiently organised or recognised to be accepted as a reliable body of knowledge or experience'.[12] If there is doubt about the expertise of a witness, this may affect the weight given to that evidence. A judge would probably not accept evidence of diagnosis and prognosis in personal injury matters from an expert other than a medical practitioner and in some cases a chiropractor.
- *Is the expert witness qualified?* The appropriate qualification may be obtained by education or by practical experience. The law is somewhat unclear as to whether the expertise can be acquired only by practical experience, but where there are no clearly established educational qualifications, practical experience has often been sufficient.

Normally a court will prefer an expert who can demonstrate that, based on the educational standards of their profession, they are accepted as an expert in their area.

Witnesses should only give evidence on matters within their area of expertise. In the case of a matter dealing with complementary medicine the use of evidence from a university or college lecturer or prominent members of a professional association with extensive practical and academic experience will likely be required. If the modality is new or not widely used, there may be difficulty in obtaining such a person, and reference to expertise from an associated modality may be necessary.

Although an expert witness is expected to be objective, there will often be disagreement among experts. This is problematic because often the disagreement will be on a matter important to the dispute at issue, such as the standard practice of the profession when faced with particular symptoms. It is for the jury or judge to draw their own conclusions as to the strength of the testimony of each expert.

What does an expert witness do?

An expert witness may become involved at an early stage in the proceedings. This will allow the expert to be involved in assessing the strengths and weaknesses of the respective cases. The involvement of the expert may include:[13]

- cooperation with the client's legal team
- preparation of a draft report for consideration by the client and legal team
- discussions on the draft report with the client's lawyer and counsel
- assisting in discovery of the opponent's documents (this means identification and recovery of relevant documents held by the other party)
- negotiations for settlement, and
- preparation of a final report for exchange with the other side.

An expert witness may be required to:

- give evidence in court based on a written report
- listen to evidence from the opposing witnesses to point out any weaknesses in the evidence, and
- be prepared to take part in negotiations with the opposing expert witnesses regarding any settlement.[14]

Giving evidence

The solicitor and barrister for the client will control the carriage of the matter. In pre-trial discussions, the expert witness should be advised of how the barrister is intending to deal with the evidence, though the witness should not be coached to provide particular answers. An expert witness should avoid the temptation to go beyond their preparation and the parameters of their report. When responding to questions, the witness should speak clearly and address the judge or jury. These behaviours rely on proper and thorough preparation for the case.[15]

The weight given to an expert witness's evidence depends on factors such as:[16]

- professional qualifications
- the degree to which the witness has first-hand knowledge of the circumstances
- the extent of their practical experience

- their eminence in the trade or profession
- the status of the evidence relied on (e.g. whether it has scientific or empirical support)
- the view taken by the judge or jury as to how thoroughly the witness has prepared, and
- the credibility of the witness, based on the quality of their report, oral evidence in chief, evidence under cross-examination, and any impression of honesty or competence.

As experts will often disagree on important issues, the ability of an expert witness to convince the court of the strength of their arguments is an important skill.

BOX 2.2

Practice tip

There are a number of matters that can assist you in providing an effective performance as a witness:

- Preparation. It is appropriate to discuss your testimony with the lawyer who is calling you as a witness. You should prepare by looking at the patient records and reviewing any written report you may have prepared for the case. A pre-trial conference with the lawyer can allow you to ask questions in order to understand how the lawyer will be approaching your evidence and what to expect in cross-examination.
- Tell the truth. You will be giving evidence on oath or affirmation. You should answer questions truthfully. Your credibility will be affected if you are untruthful on even a minor matter. For example, if asked whether you have discussed your testimony with your side's lawyer, you should say so. If asked whether you have been paid for your testimony, a good answer might be: 'I am paid for my time. My testimony is free.'
- Answer questions accurately. You should answer questions within your area of expertise. If you do not know the answer or need more information, it may be appropriate to say so. This may indicate to the court that you are acting as a professional should. If you don't understand the question, ask for clarification.
- Cross-examination. The opposing counsel will usually try to limit the weight of an expert witness's evidence. The counsel may achieve this by leading questions and other techniques such as:

    - repeating a question so as to suggest that the witness does not have sufficient grasp of their area of expertise to understand or answer the question
    - ridiculing the witness to suggest that they do not conform with the standard expected of expert witnesses, and
    - manoeuvring the witness to make an admission that will assist the counsel's client's case.

A witness should be aware of these techniques. The best means to overcome such attacks is to remain calm and to rely on thorough preparation. Becoming involved in a baiting game with the lawyer may be folly, as he or she is trained to deal with such approaches and it may not create a good impression for the court.

Format of report

The following matters should be considered by a chiropractor who prepares a report on the prognosis for a plaintiff injured, for example, in a motor vehicle accident (subject to local legal and procedural requirements):[17]

- the history of the client in relation to the injury or complaints from which the client now suffers
- the results of the examination
- any special diagnostic reports, including x-ray and pathology reports
- the prognosis for the client's condition
- whether the condition has stabilised or further deterioration could occur
- whether there is any residual disability
- whether further treatment will be required and the costs of that treatment
- the impact on current and future employment prospects in terms of the disability
- if the event is alleged to have aggravated a pre-existing condition, the degree to which this aggravation has affected the ability to work (note that a defendant is not entitled to be a perfect specimen and may be liable if a pre-existing condition is made worse by the act)[18]
- if the injury involves the loss of use of a limb or part of a body, the percentage of loss suffered, and
- if the report is from a treating chiropractor, the full details of treatment given.

Avoid the over-use of technical language that may create a barrier to communication. Explanation may be required.

Resources

C. Cook, R. Creyke, R. Geddes & I. Holloway, *Laying Down the Law*, 9th ed., Butterworths, Sydney, 2014.

J.F. Corkery, *Starting Law*, 2nd ed., Scribblers Publishing, Mudgereeba, Qld, 2002.

Notes

1 In some cases, a witness may be directed to give evidence in narrative form, rather than simply answering questions provided by counsel. See S. Odgers, *Uniform Evidence Law*, 8th ed., Thomson Reuters, Sydney, 2009, p. 95.

2 Ibid., p. 290.

3 Ibid., p. 298.

4 A. Katzmann, 'Cross-examination of the Expert Witness' in R. Winfield (ed.), *The Expert Medical Witness*, Federation Press, Sydney, 1989, p. 56.

5 Ibid., p. 41.

6 G. Hunt & A.M. Kleynhans, 'Chiropractors' Evidence', in I. Freckelton & H. Selby (eds), *Expert Witnesses*, Law Book Company, Sydney, 1993, p. 42. 420.

7 *Safety Rehabilitation and Compensation Act 1988* (Cth), s 4(1), osteopath and chiropractor; *Workers Compensation Act 1987* (NSW), s 59, chiropractor, osteo-path, masseur; *Workplace Injury Rehabilitation and Compensation Act 2013* s 3 (Vic), chiropractor and osteopaths; *Workers Compensation and Rehabilitation Act 2003* (Qld), s 7, Schedule 6, chiropractor and osteopaths; *Return to Work Act 2014* (SA), s 4, chiropractors and osteopaths; *Hup v R.O. Workers Compensation (1995)* AWCCD 74–728, naturopath treatment not compensable even though recommended by medical doctor as not performed

or supervised by medical doctor; *Workers Compensation and Injury Management Act 1981* (WA), Schedule 1 cl 17, chiropractors; *Workers Rehabilitation and Compensation Act 1988* (Tas), s 74, chiropractor and osteopath; *Workers Compensation Act 1951* (ACT), ss 2, 70, Dictionary, chiropractor, osteopath and masseur. Note the conservative views of the Workers Compensation Board of Western Australia in *Miller v Eric Roberts and Co* (1981) 1 SR (WA) 370.

8 Freckelton & Selby, *Expert Witnesses*, p. 42. 400.

9 *Amanatidis v Accident Compensation Commission* (unreported Accident Compensation Tribunal, 8 June 1990, 09/1363). In a recent case in South Australia, WorkCover Corporation (SA) did not accept expert evidence of a chiropractor: *Chiropractors Association of Australia (SA) v WorkCover* SC Doyle CJ 26/2/99, 1999, SASC 120 BC 9901075, Unreported.

10 Annotation 52 ALR 2 d 1384 (1957).

11 SASC No SCCRRM 95/593.

12 King CJ in *Bonython v R* (1984) 38 SASR 45.

13 M.P. Reynolds & P.D. King, *The Expert Witness and His Evidence*, BSP Professional Books, Melbourne, 1988, p. 7.

14 Ibid., p. 17.

15 Ibid.

16 Ibid., p. 19.

17 Winfield, *The Expert Medical Witness*, p. 10.

18 Ibid., p. 13.

3 Ethical practice and professional decision-making

Without an adherence to ethical standards, a practitioner will have little to offer a client. A professional person should be distinguished from a layperson not only by technical knowledge but also by an observance of professional ethics. Healing prospers in an environment where the health professional can be trusted for their technical skill and also for their personal honesty and respect for the client. A concern for ethical standards will help your practice to prosper, and will avoid the negative impact of disciplinary action by a statutory or professional body.

Ethical behaviour derives from a personal decision by a practitioner to act for the benefit of both the client and the profession. This decision may be based on the practitioner's personal ethical principles and/or on rules of practice specified in a code of ethics.

BOX 3.1

Action plan

- Read and understand your professional organisation's code of ethics or, if relevant, statutory rules or code of conduct.
- Treat clients and colleagues with respect and in a professional manner.
- Place your clients' interests above your own.
- Provide safe and legally compliant premises for your practice.
- Maintain professional indemnity insurance.
- Make sure that you and your professional employees are qualified and fit to practise.
- Make sure your practice is within the law and your area of expertise.
- Do not have sexual relationships with your clients.
- Respect your clients' need for privacy.
- Be honest in all matters associated with your practice.
- Make sure your practice and your professional qualifications are marketed and/or advertised legally and without misrepresentation.
- Respect your clients' confidentiality.
- Maintain accurate client records.
- Know your obligations and entitlements in the case of professional misconduct proceedings.

DOI: 10.4324/9781003195931-3

The basis of ethical conduct

Important questions for any practitioner are: What are ethics? Why should I concern myself with ethics? Isn't it enough for me to perform my professional tasks competently?

Why people act ethically

'Ethics is centrally concerned with the cultivation of moral character.'[1] Johnstone defines ethics as 'a critically reflective activity fundamentally concerned with a systematic examination of the moral life and designed to illuminate what we ought to do by asking us to consider and reconsider our ordinary actions, judgements and justifications'.[2] 'Bioethics, which involves the application of ethical principles in the context of health care and life sciences, has been described as 'the systematic study of the moral dimensions—including moral vision, decisions, conduct and policies—of the life sciences and health care, employing a variety of ethical methodologies in an interdisciplinary setting'.[3] Johnstone notes that, from her perspective as a nursing practitioner, ethical philosophy as applied to the healing professions has developed along a medico-centric model, reflecting the predominant philosophical influence.[4] There is an abundance of literature about medical ethics that contrasts with the dearth of information relevant to complementary medicine ethics. The simple application of medical ethics to complementary medicine can result in a jaundiced view of the ethics of complementary practice. The very different therapeutic approaches taken by complementary and orthodox medicine practitioners and their diverse philosophical backgrounds require an assessment of how ethical practice should be interpreted in this different context.[5]

Most people have a moral code that affects how they react to situations on a daily basis. Their idea of 'right' or 'wrong' tells them whether or not particular behaviour is appropriate. This moral code may be based on a religious tradition that supports behaviour such as telling the truth, and may suggest that taking advantage of someone is an inherently immoral act. Someone may comply with a moral code simply because they see themselves as a moral person. Others may take a more utilitarian approach, believing that moral behaviour is important for a properly functioning society, or that the cost of immoral behaviour is not worth the advantages it may bring. Unbeknownst to those applying this moral code, they may be applying some classic ethical principles, as discussed in the following sections, which provide guidance in circumstances where difficult clinical and professional decisions must be made.

Ethical dilemmas

An ethical dilemma for a health practitioner is where a practitioner is faced with a decision that requires a choice to be made between what are often unpleasant or difficult alternatives. The choice may even require breaching an ethical principle, discussed below. It is hoped this discussion about competing ethical principles and issues will assist in making these difficult decisions less difficult and more reflective of well-based ethical principles.

In orthodox medical practice, ethical dilemmas can arise frequently in regard to life-and-death decisions, for example when dealing with the wishes of family members regarding a dying relative, or whether an abortion should be carried out in the case of likely severe disability in the child. For complementary medicine, ethical dilemmas may arise over whether to accept for treatment a client who has decided to ignore medical options in an end-of-life situation when the medical treatment could extend their life. Other examples include deciding what your actions should be if you are advised by a client of the activities of another complementary medicine practitioner that appear to be dangerous or criminal in nature, or where a client is making a choice between different modalities and attaching conditions to the choice that may not be acceptable to the practitioner.

Before we deal with some of these ethical dilemmas in detail, it is appropriate to consider some of the theory of ethical practice that can assist a practitioner in deter-mining the correct ethical decision in these types of situations. For a complementary medicine practitioner, unlike in orthodox medical practice, the aim may not be to relieve symptoms but to maintain harmony in the body and focus on prevention; any healing might not occur because of a practitioner 'doing' something to the client, but rather because the practitioner and client are working as partners towards a desired outcome. Some complementary medicine practice relies primarily on traditional or empirical evidence, based upon what the practitioner and the client consider works rather than scientific evidence. In terms of the ethical obligations for a complementary medicine practitioner this might suggest a greater focus on the views of the client and client empowerment about what they are seeking with the treatment, though that will depend upon the modality.[6]

In many cases the ethical decision-making process will not be in the context of a team or group, or in a hospital setting involving different health practitioners and levels of decision-making and protocols, as may apply to some orthodox medical sit-uations; rather, it will involve an ethical decision by a sole complementary medicine practitioner. Despite these significant differences, the principles derived from bioeth-ics can provide valuable insights in the decision-making process for complementary medicine practitioners.

Ethical theories

People are the product of a particular cultural context that provides an ethical back-ground to their personal ethical stance on certain issues. This cultural morality may provide guidance about what a person might consider right and wrong, but it may not provide the tools to deal with complex decision-making in a health profession context when more sophisticated understanding of ethical decisions may be required.[7] An eth-ical dilemma may best be resolved through an understanding of well-accepted ethical theories to determine the most correct decision through a process of applied ethics. Many practitioners will, without knowing, apply these types of theories, and may recognise some of these theories in their decision-making within or outside of their professional responsibilities. These theoretical tools assist the reasoning process by identifying relevant considerations beyond reliance only on gut feelings about what is right or wrong. In this way the depth and objectivity of the process may be enhanced, including understanding ethical decisions from perspectives broader than their own. There are a number of schools of ethical thought but this text will focus on three in particular: consequentialism (which is an aspect of utilitarianism), deontology and virtue ethics.

Consequentialism

Consequentialism is an ethical theory which considers that moral rightness and wrongness depend upon the consequences of those decisions that focus particularly on creating the greatest welfare for the common good, such as reducing pain and maximising pleasure.

The motives, intention and nature of the action are basically irrelevant. In this sense this theory involves comparisons between different decisions to determine which among the outcomes that are expected to arise are likely to create the greatest benefit for the most persons under consideration. The theory might be seen as suggesting we consider the best possible consequence on a case-by-case basis, though this is not normally how decision-making is undertaken; rather, prior consideration can create rules, policies or norms derived from consequentialism that should lead to the best result in relation to overall benefit subject to exceptional circumstances. This form of utilitarianism is called rule utilitarianism.[8] An example of the application of this theory might be that respecting confidentiality is a positive thing, as without that obligation the client may not be prepared to provide the information that is required to complete competent practice or may not seek assistance at all.[9] A consequentialist perspective might suggest it is justified to assault a person at an appropriate level to protect a family member as the result justifies the action.

Deontology

Deontology does not view consequences as irrelevant but focuses primarily on the rights and duties that arise from the situation at hand. These duties may derive from religious views if the duty is considered to derive from God. This theory is normally considered to have derived from the philosopher Immanuel Kant, who spoke about the focus of ethical action based upon the Categorical Imperative and the Universal Law, which suggests that one should act based upon what should apply to all persons in a similar situation. This involves a formal or reasoned approach to ethical decision-making. It suggests, for example, that one asks 'What if everyone did what I am choosing to do?' If I decide to lie in a particular situation, if everyone did that then that would result in a breaking down of the whole concept of trust and would accordingly be wrong. The Categorical Imperative may also incorporate more specific duties such as honesty, autonomy or refraining from harming others, based upon the biblical principle of doing unto others that which you would choose to have done unto yourself. Deontology would suggest that once it is determined what your duty is in a particular context, doing your duty is always the best approach and not doing your duty is inevitably incorrect.[10]

Virtue ethics

This is a very different approach to ethics as its adherents consider the theories discussed above to focus too much on actions, while this theory focuses on character.[11] In that sense, a person applying virtue ethics considers not so much what one should do but what sort of person one should be, on the basis that a virtuous person will understand which is the right action to follow. Aristotle suggested that ethics was concerned with flourishing, based upon the basic nature of a person to achieve a good life. In the same way an animal has a natural order of living, a human being has the capacity for rational thought and this should be promoted through the application of virtues or character traits, such as honesty, generosity, courage and integrity. The bottom line is that right action comes from being a virtuous person and doing what a virtuous person would do in a particular situation. Our virtuous nature can be developed by emulating virtuous role models. It is probably correct that a well-drafted code of ethics could help in regard to virtue ethics by assisting with the cultivation of moral character and thus leading to a greater likelihood of ethical decision-making.[12]

Professional bioethics

The issue of ethics in a professional context is somewhat more complicated than in other spheres of life. A professional complementary medicine practitioner, like any professional, is in a special position based on the specialised knowledge that they 'profess' to have as a naturopath, chiropractor, massage therapist, and so on. This knowledge means that a professional is at an advantage compared with any client who might consult them. This power differential requires a balance to that power which can be found in professional ethics.

The therapeutic relationship between a practitioner and client will often emphasise an active role for the client in the prescribed treatment or therapy. Despite this, the client will rely on the practitioner's knowledge, experience and training. The client may have little idea about whether the practitioner is providing worthwhile advice or treatment, or whether the treatment has any therapeutic effect. The client will usually be asked to divulge personal information about their health and personal life and will rely on the practitioner to keep this information confidential.[13] The client may be in a vulnerable state as they have sought treatment for an ailment or illness.[14] It is this vulnerability and unequal bargaining power that are the basis of many of the ethical precepts discussed in this chapter.

The relationship between a practitioner and client will often create a positive caring relationship or friendship, through which the therapeutic impact of treatment is augmented. In this environment, 'well meaning clients and professionals alike can lose perspective of their relationship because the ordinary boundaries between private and public, secret and open, mine and thine get blurred. The appearance of intimacy can get confused with the real thing.'[15] The role of professional ethics is to provide a basis from which professionals can ascertain where their professional and personal roles diverge for the benefit of the client, the profession and the general public.

Fundamental concepts of bioethics

Beachamp and Childress suggest that there are four principles of biomedical ethics that provide 'an analytical framework intended to express general norms of the common morality that are a suitable starting point for biomedical ethics'.[16] The value of these principles is that they incorporate aspects of the ethical theories discussed above, while attempting to incorporate universal notions of morality.[17] They require a practitioner alone or in a group to determine which principle is more significant in a given situation.

The ethical theories discussed in this chapter are derived from a number of funda-mental principles:[18]

- the principle of *beneficence* (the principle of healing)
- the principle of *non-maleficence* (to refrain from causing harm, including physical, financial and emotional exploitation)
- the principle of *respect for autonomy* (this emphasises informed consent for proce-dures and allowing patients to be active in the healing process), and
- the principle of *justice*.

These principles have been criticised for not indicating how they can be reconciled when they may appear to be irreconcilable in specific factual situations.[19]

Beneficence

Beneficence is focused on the principle of helping people. The principle of beneficence may apply somewhat differently in relation to complementary medicine. For ortho-dox medicine, derived from Hippocratic tradition, the relief of suffering is a primary concern. This goal involves curing those who can be cured and caring for those who cannot.[20] A medical doctor may consider a medical intervention for an asymptomatic person to be unnecessary and unethical. A medical doctor uses allopathic techniques or other interventions to counteract symptoms through the use of pharmaceutical substances or surgical procedures. For a complementary medicine practitioner, 'curing' may be defined in different terms. The complementary medicine concept of healing, through the promotion of harmony across a patient's physical, spiritual and emotional dimensions, is foreign to orthodox medicine. A complementary medicine practitioner practising under a wellness model may perceive orthodox medicine as overly symptomatic and narrow in its approach. For a complementary medicine prac-titioner, beneficence may not require the curing of any condition. Rather, the practi-tioner may see his or her role as being to promote harmony by encouraging the client's own restorative forces to establish wellness and vitality, not simply a lack of symp-toms.[21] What is unethical or over-servicing for a medical doctor may be at the heart of the service a complementary medicine practitioner seeks to provide.

This principle requires a practitioner to consider the benefit a treatment provides as against any potential harm. From an orthodox medicine perspective, this creates an ethical dilemma for a complementary medicine practitioner who may be unable to point to scientifically based evidence of benefit or safety.[22] Orthodox medicine may demand scientific evidence of efficacy but complementary medicine may rely on tradi-tional, empirical or anecdotal evidence. Drawing on the principle of autonomy, many patients will choose a therapy with knowledge of the available level of evidence of efficacy. Some patients will rely on a personal empiricism approach—'it works for me'—and may choose to ignore evidence to the contrary. Within the culture of the complementary medicine modality, the use of this treatment would be ethical if a patient were not misled as to the nature of the treatment and evidence for benefit.[23]

Despite this perspective, if the evidence of efficacy and safety is completely absent it may be unethical to provide that treatment.[24] This would occur most clearly if there were no traditional or well-based empirical evidence to support its use. This ethi-cal concern would apply unless the client was fully informed of the lack of a valid knowledge base and indications of therapeutic benefit and that it was possible any benefits were reliant on patient perceptions of benefit or placebo.

Non-maleficence

The principle of non-maleficence requires a practitioner to avoid behaviour that negatively affects a client's interests. It is said that in orthodox medicine 'safety is sacred'.[25] Examples of a breach of this principle might be an injury suffered by a negligently applied procedure or the application of a procedure that is inherently dangerous. It could include a breach of confidence that injures a client; using an unequal bargaining position to unduly influence a client to their detriment; becoming sexually involved with a client; or a practitioner treating a client when impaired. This principle would designate as unethical the application of a treatment that harmed the client without a compensatory benefit or undertaking expensive treatment with little or no evidence or prospect of success or improvement.

Autonomy

Respect for autonomy is maintained by protecting a person's entitlement to make decisions affecting their health. One useful definition of the ethical principle is 'self rule that is free from both controlling interference by others and from certain limitations such as inadequate understanding that prevents meaningful choice'.[26] The emphasis on this aspect of ethics is based on its relevance to the primacy given to personal values and individual autonomy in Western culture.[27]

This principle is reflected in the legal concepts of consent and the requirement to advise of the risks of treatment.[28] For a complementary medicine practitioner, the obligation is emphasised when a client contemplating treatment has little or no specific or general knowledge of the nature of a modality. A practitioner should obtain consent to touch and to the modality contemplated, based upon adequate information. This point is underlined where a number of different modalities, such as massage, acupuncture and heat, are used over a number of treatments. A separate consent should be obtained at each juncture for each intervention. As complementary medicine will often rely on a partnership therapeutic relationship between the practitioner and client, where an important aspect of that relationship is self-healing promoted by the practitioner, the client's involvement in decision-making and this ethical principle is pivotal to ethical practice.

Justice

The concept of justice can be viewed from two perspectives. One perspective is as 'distributive justice', in the sense of the just and equitable distribution of benefits in society.[29] The other perspective is the ability to obtain compensation for wrongs done. The distributive aspect is reflected in the *United Nations Universal Declaration of Human Rights*,[30] which states that 'everyone has the right to a standard of living adequate for the health and wellbeing of himself [sic] and his [sic] family including medical care'.[31]

With the limited funding available for health care, should society support unproven therapies?[32] Many commentators would answer in the negative,[33] arguing that decisions about government funding should be made on the basis of scientific evidence.

This approach involves a government denying funding for treatment that is desired by a citizen, based upon the orthodox medicine therapeutic model that rejects complementary medicine as appropriate. That could be seen as a form of medical chauvinism. One solution to this dilemma is for more research to become available on the effects, costs and benefits of complementary medicine.[34] Private individuals in a just society should be entitled to choose, and to be afforded appropriate protection for that choice.

Due to government policy, complementary medicine is generally unsupported by Medicare other than for specific programs for chiropractors and osteopaths, and in relation to acupuncture by medical doctors and physiotherapists. For this reason, access to complementary medicine is primarily through the private sector. This excludes many potential clients on a financial basis, and may offend the principle of justice. The increasing coverage of complementary medicine by private health insurance broadens access to complementary medicine services, but this coverage is only available for those able to afford what is normally the maximum level of health insurance.

The principle of justice, as it relates to compensation for harm, requires consideration of the need for professional indemnity insurance. Professional associations normally require professional indemnity insurance as a requirement of membership, and will often assist members to obtain indemnity insurance though it is possible to source it individually. For non-members, professional indemnity insurance is not compulsory before practice is commenced. Some practitioners decide to avoid this obligation and risk personal liability. This decision is made by relying upon their confidence about the quality of their practice; the benevolent nature of the modality and their clients; or, more worryingly, their lack of personal assets to justify legal action against them.

The ethical issue arises here if injured clients are not able to recover compensation for loss if the practitioner does not have sufficient assets to satisfy any possible liability in negligence or contract resulting in an inability to recover compensation, which would be contrary to the justice principle. This supports substantial incentives for membership of responsible professional associations that require practitioners to obtain professional indemnity insurance.[35]

Complementary medicine without scientific evidence

Is it unethical for a practitioner to apply a technique for which there is no scientific evidence of safety?[36] Orthodox medicine may suggest that ethical practice requires the pre-market testing of materials and scientific trials for procedures to test safety. Traditional or anecdotal evidence that indicates safety over many generations could be sufficient unless there is scientific evidence to the contrary. This form of evidence is accepted as sufficient in a number of contexts, including by orthodox medicine.[37]

There is a debate about the percentage of orthodox medicine treatments that are based on good scientific evidence.[38] Even if the most optimistic figures are accepted, a significant percentage of orthodox medicine interventions lack appropriate support by scientific evidence.[39] Many complementary medicine interventions have limited high-quality research to support them. Supportive evidence of complementary medicine tends to rely upon statistical or non-double-blind research studies. The education and information process with clients should indicate how these approaches differ.[40]

The ethics of the provision of treatment by a medical doctor, or any practitioner, involves a cost/benefit analysis within the non-maleficence and beneficence concepts.[41] Treatments may be painful, have risks associated with them and involve substantial side-effects. The decision to treat involves determining whether the costs or potential risks of treatment are outweighed by the benefits. It is difficult to give full advice about risks if there is no information available on this issue.[42] If the potential harm of a complementary medicine intervention—which should be explained before the treatment— is not associated with an offsetting benefit, then the treatment may be unethical unless the client has a clear understanding of the experimental nature of the treatment.[43] Harm can include inconvenience, financial cost, physical pain and stress.[44]

What is the appropriate evidence of benefit? Much of the proof available for the efficacy of complementary medicine comes from traditional use, sometimes from many years of treatment, and anecdotal or empirical data. When dealing with an essentially harmless therapy, at least in terms of pain and physical injury, it is easier to accept that ethically this evidence will suffice.[45] This approach may also be appropriate for chronic conditions for which there are no successful orthodox medicine treatments.[46]

Orthodox medicine may consider that the same ethical principles should apply to the provision of complementary medicine but flexibility and developments in complementary medicine provides the opportunity for some useful understanding by both parties.[47] For some registered complementary medicine modalities such as chiropractic or osteopathy a more biomedical approach may be dominant where for those practitioners statutory requirements and the nature of the modality may result in close connections with orthodox medicine.[48]

Johnstone considers ethics from a post modernism perspective where ethics are:

> multi-perspective and multi-cultural (or pluralistic) in its vision and, as such, is open to a diversity of interpretation and understanding.[49]

The following comments by Beauchamp and Childress may support this flexibility when they suggest that:

> Principles, rules, obligations, and rights are not rigid or absolute standards that allow no compromise. Although 'a person of principle' is sometimes regarded as strict and unyielding, principles must be balanced and specified so they can function in particular circumstances.[50]

This allows for ethical flexibility and the acceptance of a health philosophy outside of the dominant orthodox medicine culture.[51] This moral durability may permit for complementary medicine practice a broader perspective than applied under orthodox medicine. This is in stark relief when considering differing cultural perspectives amongst diverse populations.[52] Johnstone notes that the predominant model of ethical philosophy in healing professions is medico-centric.[53] The very different therapeutic approach taken by complementary medicine and orthodox medicine practitioners requires an assessment of how ethical practice should be interpreted in this different context.[54]

Ethical protocol for complementary medicine practitioners

For more serious conditions, harm could result in preventing or delaying potentially beneficial orthodox medicine.[55] The following ethical precepts are suggested for complementary medicine practitioners in dealing with any condition, but particularly one that is of a serious nature:

• It should be ascertained whether the client has received either a medical diagnosis or treatment, and if so what the result of that diagnosis or treatment may be. Even for those who are critical of aspects of orthodox medicine, it is normally acknowledged that it has a strength in relation to diagnosis. Whether reliant upon sophisticated diagnostic equipment, or drawing upon an in-depth anatomical knowledge or long experience in differential diagnosis, an objective assessment of the relative strengths and weaknesses inherent in orthodox and complementary medicine is likely to conclude that orthodox medicine is good at diagnosis. Of course, an orthodox medicine diagnosis will be based upon the approach favoured by that form of medicine. The issue of diagnosis is important, as the role of a complementary medicine practitioner when not relying on an orthodox medicine diagnosis raises ethical issues. If no orthodox medicine diagnosis is available—and this may be of variable quality—the complementary medicine practitioner is undertaking the sole ethical responsibility for providing the client with the necessary information to make therapeutic decisions. This should bring with it the responsibility to refer to a medical doctor if the treatment does not appear to provide benefits or if there is suspicion of the involvement of another condition that the practitioner is not trained to treat. If orthodox medicine has proven ineffective or its side-effects are problematic, and the patient is seeking an alternative therapy, this should be discussed and noted.

• The practitioner should communicate what he or she thinks can be done for the client. The practitioner should give the likely therapeutic result of treatment, indicating the strengths and weaknesses of the therapy. The likely costs and length of treatment should be canvassed. The options available to the practitioner within their modality should be discussed. The evidence of safety and or efficacy supporting the therapy, or the basis of the intervention, should be discussed.

• The client should be encouraged not to abandon orthodox medicine unless they themselves determine this course of action. Note the discussion below in relation to the New South Wales and South Australian Codes of Conduct, which specifically deal with this issue (New South Wales Code, Clause 7).

• Any problems with combining orthodox medicine with the complementary medicine therapy, such as problematic drug/herb interactions, should be canvassed and addressed.

• If the malady does not respond, or the client requires therapy beyond the scope of the practitioner, a referral to a medical doctor should be made and the treatment stopped unless, having considered all the information available, the client wishes to continue and this course of action would not be harmful. This point is especially important when a therapy derives its proof of efficacy and safety from empirical or non-scientific data. If the client does not respond as expected, the treatment should be reviewed.[56] If practicable, contact or cooperation with the client's medical doctor would be preferable to avoid misunderstanding and to maximise the possibility of complementary treatment.

These criteria could be incorporated into an express contract between the practitioner and client. This protocol acknowledges the importance of communication with the client that is at the heart of ethical conduct. A client is entitled to be given sufficient information to understand what is being agreed to, and the limits and nature of the evidence for a particular therapy.[57] It is suggested that it is not ethical to provide a treatment for which there is no evidence of safety.[58] To withhold treatment in that circumstance respects a client's autonomy and complies with the ethical precepts of beneficence and non-maleficence.

A client provided with the information to make an informed choice to use complementary medicine—which may not have scientific proof of efficacy—over what may be scientifically proven orthodox medical treatment is a client choosing their autonomous path. Client autonomy requires a balancing of the beneficence/non-maleficence principle when a client requests a treatment. From an orthodox medicine perspective, provision of treatment that has not been scientifically proven is the provision of useless treatment. But clients are entitled to choose another way based on their viewpoint of what constitutes healing and what healing should be like.[59] This principle sits best in an information-rich environment in which a client appreciates the factors that should be considered in making that decision. This ethical dilemma for a complementary medicine practitioner reflects the tension that exists between being consistent with scientific method and respecting the decision of a client to use a treatment that may not be backed by scientific evidence.[60]

There are potentially significant ethical problems that can arise where a client has determined not to commence or continue orthodox medicine where those treatments have scientifically proven benefits. If a complementary medicine practitioner seeks to dissuade a client from taking advantage of those options, then the ethics of the approach could be questioned as potentially in breach of the non-maleficence precept.

Where the complementary medicine treatment does not rely on scientific evidence and is being promoted as being an alternative therapy rather than simply a complementary therapy, an ethical dilemma arises for a complementary medicine practitioner. Is this course of action in the best interests of the client? The client may, armed with the knowledge of orthodox medicine options, determine to take that course based upon their autonomous choice for many valid reasons such as spiritual beliefs, lifestyle, age and concerns about orthodox medicine's side-effects. A complementary medicine practitioner in that case has an ethical obligation to indicate the cost/benefit analysis of their therapy and the evidence of efficacy and safety of the therapy. Only then can the autonomy of the client and the ethical concepts of beneficence and non-maleficence be reconciled. The more cautious ethical procedure is to attempt complementary treatment, if this is possible.

Application of ethical theory

It is not necessary to simply apply just one theory to determine ethical behaviour, rather each of the theories discussed on pages 21–23 has important insights that can be used as tools in good ethical decision-making. By applying the essence of these theories it should become clear that outcomes are important, as are rights and the development of a virtuous character. Understanding significant ethical concepts does not guarantee practitioners will act ethically but it allows a decision-maker to take aspects of each theory to determine correct action from a number of different perspectives.

Beauchamp and Childress suggest that the following approaches can be applied to provide a sufficient and strong justification for an ethical decision, namely: (1) the moral rules, principles and theories discussed above; (2) lived experience and case examples of individual personal judgements; or (3) a synthesis of both theoretical and experiential approaches. Beauchamp and Childress prefer the third approach as the one most likely to result in the correct decision.[61]

It is important to note that the ethical theories will often conflict when considering a particular fact scenario, so it may be a process of determining which theory applies best to a particular factual situation. Other issues also impact on ethical decision-making, such as the institutional setting—for example, are you working with people of limited means; in a large practice or as a sole practitioner? Are you considering the ethical decision in the context of working with another practitioner, such as a medical doctor, chiropractor or naturopath? These types of issues may not always figure prominently in orthodox bioethics situations but they are relevant for consideration nonetheless. The contextual issues may impact on how the decision is considered and may provide an easier decision involving referral or truly complementary treatment where the complementary medicine is provided alongside medical treatment.[62]

The theories and principles discussed above appear to make decision-making complex but the application of experience and judgement, and a balancing of relevant considerations, is most likely to derive the best option, though people may differ in their views on such matters. Below is a five-step structure that might usefully be applied when determining difficult ethical issues. Note that this incorporates provision for a final justification for the decision reached to deal with the possibility that a personal view may ignore the application of other sound reasons for a particular and perhaps different result. Conscious justification of a conclusion can avoid ethically debatable decisions influenced by prejudice and self-interest and overly influenced by gut feelings, though there may be value in intuitive responses as a possible starting point in considerations.[63] Ethical decision-making involves 'evaluating moral decisions underlying health care, and is thus a conscious activity'.[64]

1 Identify and describe available options

- What are the possible courses of action based upon clinical indications?
- What are the possible intended or foreseeable outcomes from each option?
- Consider the wishes of the client?

Note that the best evidence available is essential to undertaking this process and it may provide an easier answer to any dilemma. In the context of complementary medicine practice there is a need to respect the capacity of orthodox medicine to use technology to provide a diagnosis from its perspective and provide information that can assist in decision-making without ignoring the diagnosis process from the complementary modality perspective. If any contemplated action is required or prohibited by statute, such as supplying prescription medicine, this may avoid the need to consider it an ethical dilemma and make the decision much easier.

2 What factors are suggestive of a particular option?

Applying appropriate ethical principles and theories, what reasons favour a particular option?

- Legal obligations such as Therapeutic Goods legislation, restricted acts or common law duties? (see Chapter 6)
- Beneficence—what is in a client's best interests based on their aims, goals and values?
- Non-maleficence—are any risks compensated for by the benefits? If not, is the treatment ethically justified?
- Autonomy—what does the client want to do?
- Justice—what is the most cost-effective method? What is the fairest way to proceed?
- Utilitarianism—what are the best expected consequences for everyone concerned?
- Deontology—what would happen if all persons applied this type of consideration?
- Virtue ethics—what would a good practitioner do in this situation?

3 Reasons against particular options

Applying appropriate ethical principles and theories, what reasons are against a particular option?

- Actions breaching legal obligations such as Therapeutic Goods legislation, restricted acts or common law duties?
- Beneficence—what is not in client's best interests based on their aims, goals and values?
- Autonomy—does this option go against what the client wants to do?
- Non-maleficence—does it harm the patient and is there no counter-balancing benefit?
- Justice—what is the more expensive method? What is the fairest option?
- Utilitarianism—what is the worst or less positive expected consequences for everyone concerned?
- Deontology—does it involve treating someone as a mere means?
- Virtue ethics—is it the type of thing an unethical practitioner would do in this situation?

4 Evaluate options

Compare the options based upon the above considerations.

- Identify any particularly strong or weak reasons.
- Which options should be discarded based upon the above balancing process?
- Which options are decisively indicated—is it a requirement by law or professional obligation?

5 Making the decision

- Which, on balance, is the best option?
- Justification—what makes this option the preferable option and other options less appropriate?

Examples of ethical dilemmas and possible approaches

Below are some examples of how ethical dilemmas may be resolved. These are only examples and small changes to the facts and context may result in a different result. Different perspectives may suggest another valid approach but it is hoped that these examples may provide useful guidance to ethical professional decision-making.

Case study

A client has been attending a naturopath for a number of months. The client is also under the care of a physician for depression and the naturopath, with the knowledge of the physician, has been providing advice on diet and general well-being. At one appointment the client tells the naturopath in a serious conversation that he thinks his problems are primarily caused by his wife and he thinks his best option is to assault her. The naturopath is aware that the client has a violent past with his wife and is not certain whether he will carry out his threat but the risk is real. The naturopath asks the client to urgently speak to his physician and suggests making an appointment immediately. The client says the physician is away and in any event the physician would not understand and would just report him to the police. The client says, 'Please don't tell anyone—it is our secret.' The naturopath counsels him strongly against that act and suggests seeking assistance from another physician or other mental health institution.

In terms of the ethical dimension, the question involves a consideration of three options. Option one is to not mention this to anyone on the basis he probably will not perform the threatened act. That would preserve the confidentiality of the client. Option two is to advise the wife of what has been stated. Option three is to advise the police and the wife.

Ethically there is an obligation to keep confidential information confidential for the benefit of the client. In terms of the principle of beneficence, if nothing happens, not advising of this threat may assist the client in confirming his trust for the naturopath, but the result of him acting out the threat may mean the client will commit a very serious criminal offence, which if he is convicted of this crime will involve a long prison sentence. The principle of autonomy might on one view suggest his wishes should be respected but that principle is not appropriately applied here. The application of justice would suggest primarily attention to the potential harm to a third party and applying a utilitarian viewpoint would result in damage, and potentially death, to a third party (the wife) and to the client. In terms of non-maleficence, harm would be done to the wife and client if this information was not provided to relevant authorities. On balance, in applying the fact scenario, relevant ethical principles and the fact that the client has previously indicated a violent tendency, the ethical decision in this situation would most likely be to report the threat to the police for their action. This would be justified, and would be the best and strongest ethical option based upon the issues outlined above. It would presumably result in the loss of a client, potential security issues for the naturopath in the future and the need to justify a breach of client confidentiality, but if applying virtue ethics, it would be the kind of decision an ethical practitioner would make.

Case study

You are a homoeopath with an elderly woman as a client. A close relative of the client approaches you about your client. The client has been diagnosed with advanced bowel cancer by a doctor in a major hospital. The client has not been informed because she is old and does not speak English very well. You have been treating the client for abdominal pain. The doctor and relatives think it would be devastating for her to hear the prognosis and, owing to the nature of the disease, they prefer not to tell her the worst as they do not intend to treat the client for her illness, which is likely to end in death in the near future. The relative wants you to know as it may impact on treatment but they ask you not to tell the client.

This example raises difficult ethical issues. Clearly the two options here are to accept the approach taken by the doctor and relatives or to seek to advise your client of this new information. First, it is possible to argue that this information is outside of the scope of practice for a homoeopath, but if the practitioner is aware of a medical diagnosis which would impact on the nature of the treatment it is very difficult to apply ethical practice without now considering the nature of treatment to take this information into account. A client has an entitlement under the principles of autonomy to understand the nature of treatment and their health status. As a health practitioner, advising her of this medical diagnosis would respect this principle. The relatives and doctor consider the client would find this information too confronting. This would impact on the beneficence principle if not telling a client this information meant she was left in the dark about what was happening to her in due course, though the family members consider it would have a negative effect on her. One needs to ask about the justification for the approach of the doctor and relatives and why they are taking this stance to determine what they see as being the best result for the client. It may be determined that medical treatment could have some value. Justice and the principle of autonomy would suggest the client should be informed of her diagnosis and prognosis so she can take part in the decision-making process. The likely impact on the client of telling her or not telling her needs to be understood to determine what might be the ethical approach. Are the relatives and doctors taking a paternalistic approach to the client? Is the client in a position where she is deemed not competent to understand such matters? Is not advising the client of her condition the type of thing an unethical practitioner might do?

In evaluating these options a practitioner should consider what he or she knows about the nature of the client in terms of her understanding and likely reaction to this information. If it is possible that the most ethical approach is to provide the prognosis to the client, it must be considered whether it is appropriate to speak to the family members and family doctor about your views, encouraging them to provide that information before any action is taken and to carefully consider the feelings of the client in how the information is imparted. The role of applying ethical concepts should also consider the cultural context of those decisions, as the family may take a much larger role in the decision-making process than applies in other cultural contexts. Whichever decision is made would require the practitioner to consider whether the homoeopathic treatment should continue, as the provision of treatment that may be futile would breach the justice principle and may have a financial cost and harm to the client with little gain. This consideration could include a decision to change treatment to deal with the reality of the illness being treated, but that may require revealing something of the nature of the illness.

Case study

A registered Traditional Chinese Medicine (TCM) practitioner obtains a new client who tells her she has recently attended a local practitioner newly arrived in Australia who calls himself an 'Oriental medicine practitioner'. The practitioner is not registered and he reuses acupuncture needles after he puts them in boiling water. What should the TCM practitioner do?

Option one is to advise the client strongly about the risks involved in such practice, and approach that practitioner and refer them to the breach of protected title provisions and the health risks involved. Option two would involve advising the relevant registration board; while option three would be to do nothing. Applying the concept of utilitarianism may suggest either option one or two, as this practice may cause harm to the client or another person. There is technically no obligation on a registered health practitioner to report a non-registered practitioner to the relevant board (refer to ss 140–41 National Law). It is worthwhile noting that under the current New South Wales and South Australian Codes of Conduct for Unregistered Health Practitioners and the proposed National Code of Conduct, a separate clause 4 specifically deals with the obligation to report concerns about the conduct of other health care workers.

The use of the restricted title would breach the National Law and should be reported to the relevant board. This will be for the benefit of all consumers and possibly the non-registered practitioner who may become liable if negative health outcomes arise. In this case the wishes of the client are less important but involve the public duty of the practitioner. In applying a utilitarian perspective, there is value in preventing non-qualified and apparently non-compliant and potentially dangerous practitioners from doing harm to other people, which would support an approach to the Board. This is supported by the justice principle to ensure that unnecessary injury is not caused to others. The principle of beneficence supports the reporting of this practitioner and would be supported by what an ethical practitioner would do and be part of the duty of a practitioner to deal with practitioners providing services without appropriate qualifications and most likely being misleading in their marketing.

There are few reasons not to take steps in this case, as most principles point in that direction. The practitioner should contemplate whether there is any aspect of the decision based upon self-interest in reducing competition in the marketplace. In this case the balance would suggest that taking action to report this practitioner to the Chinese Medicine Board of Australia is justified and it is suggested that the registered TCM practitioner would have an ethical duty to take that course, though not a legal obligation. Advice to the client not to undertake any treatment from the practitioner involving skin penetration is essential on legal and ethical grounds.

Case study

A naturopath prescribes vitamins and mineral supplements for a new client based upon the naturopath's assessment of the person's condition and asks the client to pay $250 for the consultation and the substances provided. The client says that as she works for a pharmacy she can get the substances or similar substances for substantially less and in addition the cost of the substances being charged is higher than that charged by other outlets in the same suburb. What should the naturopath do?

This raises a number of significant options. The options are to suggest that the client obtain the substance from another source and perhaps recommend which specific brand and quality of substance and charge only for the consultation, or provide evidence that the substances sourced from the practitioner are the only ones available that provide the quality and dosage required (if that is the case). In terms of beneficence it would be necessary to be certain that it was clinically in the best interests of the client to use the substances supplied for the price quoted. That would be justified if it could be shown that the same substance or its equivalent could not be obtained in a readily available and high-quality source for a similar or reduced price. This could more readily apply when a bespoke contemporaneous remedy was prepared by the practitioner and was not available elsewhere.

The principle of autonomy would promote the idea that a client should be provided with options to obtain substances or provided with advice that did not require purchasing expensive substances. This will require the practitioner to justify the position that a significant aspect of their compensation may be based upon profit from the sale of ingestive substances. This raises potential concerns about the conflict between the financial position of the practitioner and the financial impact on the client. If it is established that the payment for ingestive substances or their equivalent could readily be obtained by the client at a lower cost, one would doubt whether the beneficence principle and non-maleficence principle would be satisfied. That would be less problematic if the cost was the same as that available from other sources.

The other potential ethical issue is for the practitioner to consider carefully whether the ability to obtain a profit from the sale of substances had an impact on the type and amount of substances prescribed for the client, if that is the primary source of income for the practitioner. It would breach the beneficence principle and non-maleficence principle if this were to occur. The application of virtue ethics and the duty aspects of deontology would be suggestive of a duty to ensure that the interests of the practitioner and client did not conflict, which on an objective basis may possibly arise in that situation. Justification for this approach may be provided by the fact that medical doctors do not normally sell pharmaceuticals to clients and they prescribe substances dispensed by separate pharmacists, which avoids this potential dilemma from an objective basis. That is not to say that the relationship between medical doctors and pharmacy companies does not give rise to some ethical concerns. If the sale of substances by a practitioner is applied, the client should be given prior knowledge of the fact that the practitioner is receiving profit from the sale of the substance if that is the case. The best position is to apply the beneficence principle and deontology for the practitioner to charge only a service fee and prescribe substances for another outlet to dispense.

Case study

A new client attends an osteopathy clinic. The client says that she has a medical diagnosis of cancer of the colon. The client also says that she does not believe in orthodox medicine but would like to have osteopathy to deal with the cancer.

The osteopath has doubts about the treatment using osteopathy and excluding orthodox medicine. What should the osteopath do?

The issue of treatment of persons who have serious illness and the provision of complementary medicine is complicated and rife with legal and ethical issues. Drawing upon deontology, an osteopath as a registered practitioner has an obligation to recognise and work within the limits of a practitioner's competence and scope of practice (AHPRA Code of Conduct clause 1.2).[65] It is unlikely that an osteopath would consider their scope of practice would include treating cancer. That does not mean an osteopath cannot treat a client who has cancer. The options here are for the osteopath to simply state that this illness is outside of their scope of practice and not provide treatment, and to counsel the client to continue with medical options. The osteopath could, however, decide not to treat the cancer but assist with the symptoms of the disease or any side-effects of treatment. This would suggest the need for very clear information of the limitations of the services provided by the osteopath and confirmation that the osteopath is not treating the cancer but providing greater harmony in the body or treating symptoms that osteopaths normally treat. It would be important in protecting the interests of the client and in reflecting the beneficence principle and non-maleficence principle to never indicate that medical treatment should not be attempted and in fact strongly counselling the client to consider the medical option. It is suggested in terms of protecting the autonomy of the client that they are entitled to choose not to have medical treatment, if they are making that decision based upon a sound understanding of their options for treatment and the likely side-effects, outcomes and risks that arise from those options (including the risk of not undertaking that option). That is the entitlement of the client. It is justified that, based upon the beneficence principle and non-maleficence principle, the limits of the treatment for cancer by osteopathy should be thoroughly considered and discussed with the client prior to entry into treatment. This would respect the utilitarian aspect in that the best outcome for the client would most likely be attained and it is arguably the route suggested for an ethical practitioner under the virtue ethics perspective.

Case study

A client attends a chiropractic clinic where the chiropractor prefers a wellness approach to practice and does not wait for pain or disability to develop but asks clients to return every six to eight weeks to obtain chiropractic treatment. The client wants the treatment only when he feels pain, which might be once every six months or so. The chiropractor thinks this type of treatment is not in the best interest of the client as it does not provide ongoing best function. What should the chiropractor do?

One option for a chiropractor is to consider whether to accept the client on that basis. If the chiropractor does not consider this is the best option for the client and does not address the health issues involved, it may be best for the client and the practitioner to refer to another practitioner who may provide that type of service. Using a virtue ethics approach, that is what an ethical practitioner may do if they consider that the wellness approach is the appropriate practice model and, in the utilitarian sense, would result in a positive outcome from the perspective of the client. This decision could be justified as it will respect the autonomy of the client and respect the benefi-cence principle and non-maleficence principle from the perspective of the client.

Many chiropractors are more flexible in their approach and are open to different forms of treatment, and they may be prepared to accede to the request involving a non-wellness approach to treatment. The issue of what is an appropriate style of treatment may be a matter of debate. In any event, drawing on deontology principles, AHPRA Code of Conduct clause 3.1 is suggestive that in obtaining financial consent that may arise under a wellness approach or agreement for treatment contracted over a period of time, it must be based upon firm professional criteria and must not be such as to suggest over-servicing. It would be a breach of the beneficence principle and non-maleficence principle if treatment was provided at considerable cost that was not required and the condition could have been dealt with on another basis. The concept of virtue ethics suggests the need to ask what an ethical practitioner would do in this situation.

In all the above case studies the advice given to clients, and the basis of decisions made, should be recorded on the client file and, in appropriate cases, communicated directly to the client or their carer in case the matter becomes the focus of external review and the practitioner is asked to justify their decision or advice.

Codes of ethics

Professional associations for registered and unregistered practitioners and the Australian Health Practitioner Regulation Agency (AHPRA) have developed codes of conduct or codes of ethics to regulate the activities of practitioners. While a code of conduct sets out a prescribed set of moral rules and expectations for ethical pro-fessional decision-making, these are not ethics *per se*, though a well-drafted code of ethics will incorporate a useful guide to ethical conduct.[66] Practitioner members are obliged to comply with the terms of the code or risk disciplinary action in relation to a breach of the code, which can lead to suspension or exclusion from membership.

Unlike registered professions, non-registered professions have more limited stat-utory backing for their codes of ethics. Although some conduct may have civil and criminal consequences, the direct professional impact is limited to disciplinary pro-ceedings, including at worst exclusion from the organisation. For registered health professionals such as chiropractors, a practitioner found liable in disciplinary pro-ceedings may be cautioned, reprimanded, fined, suspended or have their registration cancelled.

In most states, a breach of professional ethics may result in the practitioner being subject to investigation by a health care complaints body. The power of those bod-ies to discipline practitioners is limited. A health care complaints body may refer the matter to the police in the case of criminal behaviour or to a relevant registra-tion board where an unqualified practitioner has performed a restricted act such as high-velocity cervical spine manipulation. New South Wales, Queensland, Victoria and South Australia have enacted their version of the National Code of Conduct for Unregistered Health Practitioners provides, significant remedies for breaches of the Code of Conduct provisions (refer to pages 82–92).

For chiropractors, osteopaths and Chinese medicine practitioners, a code of con-duct and other relevant policies and guidelines can be found on the AHPRA website at www.ahpra.gov.au.

Purposes of a code of ethics

Codes of ethics can take many forms. Some are very general, containing broad parameters for conduct, while others supply very detailed rules for behaviour. Many contain elements of each. The factors supporting the preparation and enforcement of codes of ethics are outlined below.

- *Professional profile.* If a profession is aware of its ethical and legal obligations, this provides benefits to all members of the profession, their clients, other professionals and the general public. If a profession is perceived as caring, professional and competent, this will increase demand for its services. A code of ethics expresses publicly the commitment of a profession to moral behaviour in a professional capacity.[67]
- *Political lobbying.* An association representing a large proportion of practitioners that enforces professional standards will be in a better position to lobby government bodies and make influential submissions to inquiries and ministers in relation to the formulation of government policy.
- *Creating awareness among the profession.* A code of ethics can motivate professionals to think about ethics and their responsibilities to a client. Codes of ethics can systemise the ethical rules of a profession, and clarify the requirements for ethical practice. A properly drafted code can provide guidance to a professional regarding what is expected of them.[68] A code of ethics can also assist in determining what is acceptable practice in the context of a negligence action or professional disciplinary proceeding.

Typical issues covered by codes of ethics

A competently drafted code of ethics can provide a helpful overview of most important ethical considerations for a practitioner. It is not intended to describe each provision of every code, but rather to highlight and comment on a number of provisions typically found in these codes.

BOX 3.2

Practice tip

Read and understand your code of ethics. This should provide an outline of your obligations, duties and entitlements as a professional. If you don't understand some aspects, seek clarification from your association. If you don't like parts of it, or think it is lacking in any way, lobby to have it changed.

Professional conduct

Conduct with clients and other practitioners

Most codes of ethics provide that practitioners should conduct themselves with clients and practitioners in a professional manner. A well-formulated code of ethics will tell a professional how to satisfy this provision.

The reputation of a practitioner will be based on factors such as:

*   the technical quality of their treatments
*   the quality of the therapeutic relationship between practitioner and client, and
*   the respect with which they are viewed by their colleagues.

The membership of a profession should bring with it collegial support, education and guidance. An important part of the education of a professional is the mentoring and advice that can come from a more experienced practitioner who has dealt with similar issues in practice.

Criticism of other practitioners

The mutual support and encouragement of colleagues should accompany membership of a profession. It may be tempting to criticise a colleague for their professional performance or in relation to their personal life. However, this temptation should be resisted for several reasons:

*   It will not engender collegial relationships with the specific practitioner or among the profession generally.
*   The practitioner may be defamed, creating liability for damages or involvement in expensive, stressful and time-consuming litigation.
*   It brings the profession into disrepute generally (criticising one member of a profession undermines the integrity of all members of the profession).
*   It may constitute professional misconduct.

If a practitioner has legitimate reservations about the professional performance or capacity of another practitioner, the options are to:

*   seek the assistance of the relevant professional association
*   refer the matter to the relevant registration board and/or health complaints body, or
*   approach the practitioner personally.

In spite of these warnings, you are still obliged to be honest in your evaluation of a practitioner's performance when acting as a witness in court or when reviewing a publication for a journal.

One significant legislative reform that applies with regard to registered health professionals, including chiropractors, osteopaths and Chinese medicine practitioners, is the mandatory notification obligations placed upon registered health practitioners and employers under the National Law (ss 140–143). Registered health practitioners and employers are obliged to notify the relevant registration board where a registered health practitioner or an employer in regard to an employee has formed a reasonable belief that a registered health practitioner has acted in a way that constitutes 'notifiable conduct'. Notifiable conduct is defined in section 140, and includes that the registered health practitioner:

*   was under intoxication by alcohol or drugs while practising or training in the profession

- has engaged in sexual misconduct in connection with the practice or training of the profession
- has an impairment that places the public at risk of substantial harm, or
- was involved in a significant departure from accepted professional standards that places the public at risk of harm.

Refer to page 64 for further details of notifiable conduct. Note that a registered health practitioner or employer may be deemed to have acted unethically in not reporting another health professional if they have formed the view that notifiable conduct has occurred. Registered health professionals and employers are protected from liability for such notifications made in good faith (refer to National Law, s 237). There is also provision for voluntary notification of less serious legal or ethical breaches (refer to National Law, ss 143 A–145).

Professional development

The standard of care expected of a practitioner will be influenced by what the profession regards as competent practice. Accordingly, it is vital to keep abreast of professional developments in ethics, technical information and administrative issues such as health fund requirements. A professional cannot maintain the standard of service necessary for optimal success without a commitment to continuing professional education. A professional who maintains interest in continuing professional education will provide a better, more up-to-date service to clients. Many professional associations require members to undertake continuing professional development as a condition of membership. One requirement for registered health practitioners under the National Law (s 128) is to undertake continuing professional development.

The health of the client

Health of the client comes first

Practitioners should avoid making professional decisions based on discriminatory grounds, or for personal reasons of convenience or financial advantage. Professionals should not take advantage of any client by using their position of influence or technical knowledge. This is fundamental to the ethical obligation of a professional. A client's lack of knowledge of the practitioner's profession requires a high degree of integrity in all dealings, to ensure that treatment and advice conform to this ethical precept.

Non-discrimination

In the provision of goods and services, federal, state and territory legislation stipulates that a person should not be discriminated against on the basis of a number of grounds, including:

- race
- gender
- impairment or disability
- age

- association
- lawful sexual activity
- marital status
- religion
- industrial activity
- responsibilities as a carer
- pregnancy.

Each jurisdiction has similar but not identical legislation. Practitioners should refer to the legislation in their own jurisdiction or seek specific legal advice, as not all the above grounds apply in all jurisdictions. Some general comments can be made.[69]

These statutes, including the *Anti-Discrimination Act 1977* (NSW), *Anti-Discrimination Act 1991* (Qld) and *Equal Opportunity Act 2010* (Vic), are breached where there is a connection between the specified grounds of discrimination and the refusal to supply or a different supply of goods and services. In many instances, the necessity of avoiding discrimination is self-evident. For example, a practitioner would clearly breach the legislation if he or she refused employment or the provision of treatment to a person on the basis of their race or religion.

More difficult issues arise where the practitioner chooses to limit the provision of services for a personal reason, such as personal security or preference, and this has the effect of discriminating against a section of the community. For example, is it a discriminatory act for a female massage therapist to limit services to female clients only because she is uncomfortable about providing services to male customers due to security issues? It might be possible to argue that the exemption relating to workplace health and safety might apply in this case, but this potentially could be considered a breach of the legislation. Although the practitioner may consider that there are good reasons for this policy, only a specific exemption from this legislation would protect a practitioner when taking this approach. Some legislation, such as section 113 of the *Anti-Discrimination Act 1991* (Qld) and sections 89–90 of the *Equal Opportunity Act 2010* (Vic), does permit application for specific exceptions to the legislation in some cases. A practitioner who seeks to practise in a manner that may exclude the provision of services to one gender should seek clarification from the relevant state anti-discrimination office.

As a general rule, it is not permissible to refuse treatment on the basis of a person's health status; however, it is normally permissible to refuse services to protect the public health, to protect the health and safety of people at a place of work or to conform with the requirements of a statute. For example, a practitioner might refuse to massage a person with a skin infection if the service would be likely to spread the infection to the detriment of public health or if the legislation requires the refusal of treatment in that situation, as is contemplated in section 48 of the *Disability Discrimination Act 1992* (Cth) and sections 106–108 of the *Anti-Discrimination Act 1991* (Qld).

Safe, hygienic premises

This obligation is reflected in health regulations administered by state and local governments. Some codes prescribe the necessity of providing toilets, washroom facilities and separate waiting areas. Some of these requirements may be difficult to satisfy for a practice operated from a residential address. Refer to some more specific comments in relation to certain types of premises at pages 203–207.

Non-injury

Clearly, practitioners should do nothing that will injure their client, either physically or emotionally. Clients should be advised that part of the healing process might involve a temporary worsening of symptoms (a healing crisis). Any risks of treatment should be fully canvassed with a client. This ethical precept is based on the ethical principle of beneficence (helping) and autonomy, which should be the ultimate goal of all healing endeavours.

Professional indemnity insurance

One purpose of professional indemnity insurance is to secure compensation for a client who has suffered damage as a result of a negligent act by a practitioner. Without such a policy, the client will seek recourse to the possibly insufficient assets of a practitioner to satisfy any judgement or settlement figure. It is a breach of the ethical principle of justice to practise when a client is effectively excluded from obtaining compensation from injury. The policy should provide an indemnity for the practitioner if the insurance company satisfies the claim made against the practitioner where the requirements of the policy have been satisfied.

   For these reasons, a practitioner should always maintain a current professional indemnity insurance policy. Most professional associations provide group policy coverage, or a practitioner should seek their own indemnity policy if they are not a member of a professional association (for more details, refer to Chapter 8).

Fitness for practice

A practitioner should not practise unless they are physically and mentally capable, and free from the influence of drugs or alcohol. A client will be placed at risk if all necessary physical and mental faculties are not available for his or her care. The standard of care applied in an action for negligence is based on the capacities of an unimpaired practitioner. A practitioner who lacks these capacities may increase his or her exposure to liability for negligence and may void the coverage provided by professional indemnity insurance. A practitioner or employee with drug or alcohol problems should obtain treatment immediately, before harm to a client and/or the reputation of the practice occurs. Even the suggestion of alcohol on the breath may raise the question of whether the practitioner is in a fit state to practise. For this reason, it is advisable not to consume alcohol or take drugs or medicines that may impact adversely on professional performance for a number of hours prior to and during practice hours.

   A registered healthcare practitioner who has a mental or physical impairment that detrimentally impacts upon their ability to practise their profession may be denied registration under the National Law or may have conditions imposed in regard to their practice.

Practising only within a discipline

A practitioner may, with appropriate qualifications, training and experience, broaden his or her professional scope and thereby improve the service provided to a client, but the following should be understood:

- *Practising outside your discipline may void the professional indemnity insurance policy.* A professional indemnity insurance policy may protect against liability for the primary activity of a profession, but not activities outside the normal scope of professional practice. For example, a massage therapist may be covered for therapeutic massage but not for acupuncture or prescribing herbs. A practitioner should understand the activities covered by their professional indemnity policy. Limiting oneself to an area of practice for which a practitioner is qualified and experienced is the best way to avoid liability for malpractice. One aspect of good professional practice is knowing your limitations. A practitioner should stay within the areas of practice for which he or she has adequate training. A practitioner could seek an extension to their insurance policy to cover that additional practice if they can demonstrate appropriate training and/or qualifications for that expanded practice.
- *Practising outside your discipline may breach environmental planning provisions.* For example, if local authority planning consent has been granted to practise chiropractic or acupuncture on the premises, it may not allow for other activities, such as the sale of herbal medicines.
- *Practising outside your discipline may breach the lease.* The commercial lease use clause may be limited to a specific professional description, such as 'homoeopathy clinic'. When negotiating a lease, include a wide usage clause to allow some room for variation in professional practice over time and the ability to assign the lease to another practitioner without having to broaden the usage clause (refer to Chapter 8).
- *It is important to refer a client to another practitioner if their condition is outside your area of expertise or skill.* Understanding your limitations is an important professional skill. If a client has a complaint that is best dealt with by a medical doctor or another practitioner, a referral should be made readily and promptly.

Sexual relationships with clients

The establishment of a sexual relationship with a client is specified as a breach of professional ethics in virtually all codes of ethics. The unequal power position inherent in professional relationships means that such activity should be avoided because it may harm the client, as well as prejudice the objectivity of advice given.[70]
    A sexual relationship with a client should be avoided for the following reasons:

- It brings the profession into disrepute.
- It is a breach of trust.
- It violates the role of the therapist.
- It may involve exploitation of a vulnerable client.
- It may impair the healing process.
- It could constitute misuse of power.

A sexual relationship with a client is a serious breach of professional ethics for medical doctors, providing grounds for deregistration or other severe sanction. A similarly strict approach should apply for complementary medicine practitioners. The concern that arises with this type of behaviour is the difficulty in maintaining professional boundaries between the client and the health professional, and the risk that could arise for a misuse of the power imbalance between a client and a health professional.

Note that it may not be considered ethical to commence a sexual relationship with a client (including family members of the client) even if the person is no longer a client. The most liberal approach to this issue would be to require a substantial gap between the cessation of the therapeutic relationship and the commencement of the personal relationship. Some would consider that even if a gap were observed, this would still not make the relationship ethical. Each case will depend on its own factors, but relevant considerations also include the strength and duration of the professional relationship; whether the client is under eighteen years of age; whether the client has a disability or disorder, including psychological disorders affecting their judgement; whether there was social contact before the professional and sexual relationship commenced; and whether the practitioner was aware the client had been sexually abused in the past. If the professional is practising in a small community, this may be a factor in determining ethical behaviour. In summary, it is best to avoid sexual relationships with clients or to observe very strict protocols when this step is contemplated.

Clause 4.9 of the Codes of Conduct for the registered professions TCM, chiropractic and osteopathy suggest that good practice involves a maintenance of professional boundaries and not using a professional position to establish or pursue a sexual, exploitative or otherwise inappropriate relationship with anybody under a practitioner's care. It notes that sexual and other personal relationships with people who have previously been a practitioner's patients or clients are usually inappropriate and this may extend beyond the completion of the therapeutic relationship. This type of approach should be applied to both unregistered and registered health professionals. The Osteopathy Board of Australia's Sexual and Professional Boundaries: Guidelines for Osteopaths (April 2013) provides a further useful discussion of the issues in this area for all health professionals.[71]

Sexual harassment

In most jurisdictions, anti-discrimination legislation penalises sexual harassment. Examples are sections 118 and 119 of the *Anti-Discrimination Act 1991* (Qld); section 22A of the *Anti-Discrimination Act 1977* (NSW) and section 85 of the *Equal Opportunity Act 1995* (Vic). Sexual harassment includes, but is not limited to, unwelcome behaviour of a sexual nature in circumstances in which a reasonable person, having regard to all the circumstances, would have anticipated that the other person would be offended, humiliated or intimidated. This would include making unsolicited demands or requests for sexual favours; inappropriate disrobing or inadequate draping; intimate examination without informed consent (this could also constitute criminal sexual assault, and would be difficult to justify for a complementary medicine practitioner); irrelevant discussion of a client's or practitioner's sexual problems or orientation; requesting irrelevant details of sexual history; conversations about the sexual fantasies of the practitioner; or making suggestive comments about a client's appearance or body.

A practitioner who follows proper professional practice would normally avoid these behaviours. If any therapy involves procedures that might trespass into these areas, a practitioner should consider whether such practices are appropriate, or should be in a position to justify that activity on well-based professional grounds.

Indecent exposure

Sensitive attention to the issue of disrobing is important for all practitioners. Any activity that unnecessarily discomforts a client should be avoided. Refer to Chapter 7, which discusses appropriate procedures for disrobing in the context of massage therapy.

The basic rules should be:

*   Limit the disrobing of clients to the minimum necessary for treatment.
*   Justification for touching must be based squarely on well-accepted professional requirements.
*   Make sure that the physical layout of premises respects clients' privacy requirements.

Explain the necessity for disrobing and any need for physical contact with the client as early as possible in the consultation. This is important, especially when a client may not expect physical contact. For example, physical contact usually would be contemplated in any massage treatment but not in a consultation for naturopathy. It is advisable to continue to communicate with the client while the service or consultation proceeds to ensure that they consent to any further stage of disrobing or physical contact, are comfortable with the process and have given consent freely. A practitioner should, as far as possible, ensure that an information-rich environment is created to allow free and open decision-making by the client.

A cautious practitioner would avoid touching intimate parts of a client's body altogether, as the possibility of misunderstanding is obvious. If a complaint of sexual assault or professional misconduct is made, although the onus of proving the charge would be on the complainant, the professional and personal ramifications of such proceedings may be serious. The determination of guilt or innocence may simply depend on who is believed by the relevant disciplinary body or court.

Place the onus on the client to disrobe to the extent to which they feel comfortable. If the practitioner considers that it is not possible to properly provide the service without disrobing beyond the point where the client is comfortable, the options are to vary the treatment or not treat the client at all.

Personal honesty

A practitioner should be honest in dealings with clients, medical benefits funds, insurance companies, colleagues and government departments. A practitioner may be tempted, at the urging of a client, to transfer professional services from one member of a family to another to overcome a limit prescribed by a medical fund. It may be tempting to provide a false certificate for workers' compensation purposes. These acts are fraudulent, and may result in criminal prosecution, professional misconduct proceedings or negative publicity about the professionalism of the practitioner and the profession.

High ethical standards should be maintained in both the professional and personal life of the practitioner. Honesty should extend to discussions about the prospects of improvement in a person's condition.

Conflict of interest

It is fundamental to the role of a profession that a practitioner avoids circumstances where his or her interests are in conflict with those of a client. This might occur where a practitioner owns a retail business attached to a professional practice and a client is pressured to purchase herbs, foods, vitamins or other substances from that business and is not given the option to purchase the product elsewhere or provided with information about where these substances can be sourced. This concern is emphasised if equivalent and cheaper sources are available to the client elsewhere. In these situations, the practitioner is obtaining financial or other benefit from the sale of products associated with the professional services. A practitioner is well advised to ensure that a client is informed that a profit will be made from the sale of any substances prescribed by the practitioner. If there are other sources for that product, they should be given the option to buy from those outlets. This may not apply to a substance such as a homoeopathic remedy that is tailored to a client's needs and may not be available for purchase elsewhere.

A conflict of interest could also occur where a practitioner obtains a financial or other benefit for the referral of a client to another practitioner.

Honest advertising

Most codes of ethics contain some controls over advertising. These normally deal with advertisements on social media or a website, and in newspapers, telephone directories, on radio and television, and in stationery.

Statutes such as the Commonwealth *Competition and Consumer Act 2010* and various state *Fair Trading Acts* affect the type of advertising permissible by professionals. These statutes penalise false and misleading advertising in relation to the provision of goods and services. Refer to the discussion below regarding the impact of consumer legislation in relation to misleading and deceptive behaviour at pages 154–164.

A professional association has a legitimate interest in attempting to limit inappropriate, misleading or unprofessional advertising by its members. Advertising is an important interface between the general public and the profession. Maintaining high standards in advertising helps develop a positive public image.

The following provisions in codes of ethics might be deemed anti-competitive and thereby unenforceable unless supported by statute. In each case, it is necessary to consider how the provisions are actually applied in the market for the services involved, and whether there is a blanket prohibition or merely regulation of an activity:

*   controls limiting advertisement of content, such as not permitting advertising other than location and specialities
*   a prohibition on advertising without approval or within approved parameters
*   a prohibition on comparison advertising
*   a prohibition on touting
*   a prohibition on advertising unless commencing or moving practice, and
*   controls on signage.

The following provisions would probably not be considered anti-competitive:

*   a prohibition on title or descriptions to suggest a qualification to which the practitioner is not entitled

- requirements that an advertisement is truthful and not in breach of the law
- limits on the use of a logo of a professional association
- requirements that advertising not be improper, exploitative or contrary to the interest of the profession, and
- requirements that advertising in relation to fees be accurate with disclosure of conditions attached.

Advertising of specialities or special expertise may affect the expected standard of care by requiring performance commensurate with that specialty. For example, if a practitioner advertises a specialisation in difficult cases or sporting injuries, this may be a factor in determining that a higher standard of care should apply. The practitioner needs to balance this risk with the marketing advantage of this type of advertising.

Registered complementary health practitioners are subject to specific guidelines in relation to advertising. With regard to chiropractors, refer to the Guidelines for Advertising of Regulated Health Services at https://www.chiropracticboard.gov.au/Codes-guidelines. aspx. (accessed 13 December 2021) For osteopaths, refer to the Guidelines for Advertising of Regulated Health Services at https://www.osteopathyboard.gov.au/Codes-Guidelines. aspx. (accessed 13 December 2021) For Chinese medicine, refer to the Advertising Guidelines for Registered Chinese Medicine Practitioners at http://www.chinesemedi-cineboard.gov.au/Codes-Guidelines.aspx. (accessed 13 December 2021)

Based upon the terms of section 133 of the National Law, a registered health professional should not advertise in a manner that is false, misleading or deceptive, or likely to be so. In addition, the advertising should not offer a gift or discount or other inducement to use the service unless the terms of the offer are specified in the advertisement. The use of testimonials is not permitted, nor are claims that create an unreasonable expectation of beneficial treatment or encourage indiscriminate or unnecessary use of the health service. These types of considerations are advisable for all professional health practitioners and provide useful information about the use of titles and qualifications in advertising. Refer to a discussion of these advertising guidelines below at pages 46–49 and 166–167.

Unusual treatments

Some codes of ethics state that, when advising a client of options for treatment, the client should be advised if the treatment is not within the generally accepted standard of practice. A claim of negligence made against a health professional will be assessed against the standard of what is widely accepted as competent professional practice by a significant number of respected practitioners in the field. A client can expect to be given information about treatment options, especially when the practitioner is suggesting a less orthodox approach. Great care should be taken by a practitioner if the treatment provided is outside of normal practice for a profession.

Titles suggesting health practitioner qualifications

The National Law (ss 113–120) provides that no person should hold themselves out (represent or advertise themselves) or use protected titles that suggest they have qualifications or registration status they do not hold. Specific protected titles are applicable solely to certain registered practitioners. Substantial penalties may apply for a breach of these provisions. For more details, see Chapter 4.

Some health practitioners use the term 'doctor'. See Chapter 7 for a detailed discussion of this point. It is essential that a practitioner ensures that, in advertising, signage, stationery and communications with clients, a practitioner is not held out as a medical doctor or other registered health professional by using a protected title. Practitioners who hold themselves out as having qualifications that they don't hold may also be liable for action under the consumer protection provisions of the Commonwealth *Competition and Consumer Act 2010* (see pages 156–161).

Claims of cures

Most codes of ethics provide that a practitioner should not claim a cure for any illness or malady. This is included to avoid outlandish claims by practitioners that, if not justified, may bring the whole profession into disrepute. It may be an illegal anti-competitive act to stop a practitioner making a claim that he or she can effect a cure. Indeed, it may be a justifiable competitive tactic by a professional to claim a cure for an ailment *if that is in fact what the practitioner is able to do.*

A practitioner should be very cautious about making such claims, as a promise to cure a complaint will probably create a contract with a client who enters treatment on the basis of that claim. The practitioner may be subject to an action of breach of contract and damages if the cure is not effected. An inability to effect a cure may leave a client angry, disappointed and distrustful, and this creates fertile ground for litigation.

A claim to cure an illness may require substantiation; otherwise a practitioner may be exposed to action by a disgruntled client or a regulator. Some persons who have made claims of miracle cures have been the subject of action under consumer legislation (refer to the discussion in Chapter 6).

In New South Wales, Schedule 3 of the Public Health Regulation 2012 provides a Code of Conduct for Unregistered Health Practitioners. Clause 5 states:

1   A health practitioner must not hold himself or herself out as qualified, able or willing to cure cancer and other terminal illnesses.
2   A health practitioner may make a claim as to his or her ability or willingness to treat or alleviate the symptoms of those illnesses if that claim can be substantiated.

The same provision is found in clause 4 of the South Australia, Queensland and Victorian Unregistered Health Practitioners Code of Conduct. Unfortunately, other than referring to 'cancer', a definition of 'terminal illnesses' is not provided. This means that a practitioner should not suggest he or she can cure the illnesses quoted in (1) but may make a claim to treat or alleviate symptoms if such a claim can be substantiated. Great care should be taken to ensure that a breach of this provision does not occur. It is suggested that, when dealing with cancer and serious illnesses, the need to keep clear and complete records of treatment given, advice provided to the client and outcomes is essential. Refer to pages 82–92 for more details of this Code of Conduct.

Claims of secret methods

If a practitioner develops or discovers a new safe and exclusive method of treatment, they are entitled to use that method for the benefit of their clients. If the method is revolutionary in nature with clear therapeutic benefits, a professional may consider that they have a responsibility to allow other practitioners to use a similar technique for the benefit of the profession and the health of their clients.

Refer to the comments above about the potential liability for false and misleading advertising or claims made in relation to the nature and quality of treatment. This type of claim may attract the attention of consumer protection bodies, who will be concerned to ensure consumers are not misled about the quality of the treatment or goods offered. Refer to Regulation 9 of the Therapeutic Goods Advertising Code Instrument 2021 which includes statements that advertising in relation to therapeutic goods must ensure any claims made in advertising are valid and accurate; not exaggerating product efficacy or performance; not suggesting that the therapeutic goods are infallible, miraculous or a sure cure.

Confidentiality

Clear and honest communication is fundamental to the healing process. A practitioner needs to establish an environment where clients are prepared to reveal and discuss the physical and emotional aspects of their health. Without a good level of communication and trust, the quality of the therapeutic relationship may be prejudiced.

The obligation to respect the client's confidence is found in most codes of ethics. A breach of this obligation may constitute professional misconduct and affect the reputation of the profession.

A duty of confidence may be an implied term of the contract between practitioner and client. Probably more significant is the requirement for confidentiality integrated into the general duty of care of a complementary medicine practitioner. In addition to these common law principles, the provisions of the Commonwealth *Privacy Act 1988* are applicable to complementary health practitioners. A discussion of this statute is provided below.

Establishment of duty of confidence

The common law duty of confidence arises in the following situations:

- *Where the information imparted to a practitioner has the quality of confidential information.* For example, most details of past medical or health history, personal circumstances and treatment would be of a confidential nature. Confidentiality will normally be implied by the circumstances without the need for any express statement by the client. Some information may not be confidential as it is public knowledge, such as a name or telephone number, though a cautious practitioner should only reveal these details to an authorised person. Practitioners should even keep confidential the fact that a particular person is a client. A client may consider the fact they are being treated for any reason to be a confidential matter.
- *Where the information is imparted in circumstances importing an obligation of confidence.* If confidential information is imparted to a practitioner in a social situation where no professional relationship exists, a legal duty of confidence may not apply. This might occur where a person talks to a practitioner at a social function about their illness or injury. The point at which a professional relationship is established may be difficult to pinpoint. Even when confidential information is revealed in a social situation, a practitioner should respect that

person's confidence. This will avoid any negative professional consequences that could result from revealing this information, even if no technical breach of the duty of confidence has occurred.

The duty of confidence covers information given orally, and would include records compiled in relation to the treatment of a client.[72] The duty of confidence survives the termination of the therapeutic relationship, and even the death of the client.[73]

Breach of duty of confidence

A breach of the duty of confidence arises where there has been an unauthorised use of confidential information to the detriment of the party who communicated that confidential information. Liability can arise even if there is no proven economic detriment to the client.

BOX 3.3

Practice tip

Breaches of confidence can occur inadvertently. There is an old saying that 'a waiting room has ears'. Clinic design should take into account the fact that clients waiting for treatment may hear the activities of the practitioner and/or employees while dealing with clients on the telephone and in person. A client may be unhappy to reveal to all the persons in the waiting room the details of their particular complaint. Even if such breaches of confidence do not generate any legal action, they may affect your reputation among those who are in earshot and the clients whose details are openly discussed. Note that communications via email or mobile phones may not be secure, and inadvertent breaches of confidence may occur.

Persons who are entitled to receive confidential information are the client, a parent of a client who is a minor (not old enough to provide a valid consent), or another person such as a member of the family or other practitioner expressly or by implication authorised to be given this information. Staff need training in the duty of confidentiality, as a practitioner may be liable for an employee's breach of confidence.[74]

Justification for breach of confidence

The duty of confidence is not absolute, and there are some situations where disclosure may be justified:

- *Expressed or implied consent by the client.* A client may expressly consent to information being revealed to a third party—for example, another professional, parent or relative, employer or insurance company. A client will normally give implied consent to information being revealed to another practitioner involved in a partnership necessary for treatment of the person. This implication would likely apply where the client consents to being referred to another practitioner—for example, a chiropractor referring a client to a naturopath. Discussions with relations or family members of a client should be undertaken only with consent, especially when the information revealed is sensitive. Consent would normally be implied where information is prepared expressly for the purpose of delivery to a third party—that is, for an employer sickness certificate or to an insurance company as part of a client's claim for injury.

The duty of confidence would apply to information supplied by a child with capacity—that is, a child over sixteen years or less than sixteen years old with the capacity to give consent (refer to pages 130–131 for details of requirements for consent obtained from minors). Consent should be obtained before disclosure of confidential information to a parent of that child.

* *Subject to order of court or tribunal.* On rare occasions, a practitioner may be required to disclose confidential information under an order of a court or tribunal. Information supplied by a client to their lawyer is privileged and need not be revealed, even to a court. Complementary medicine practitioners do not enjoy that special privilege. A practitioner may be deemed to be in contempt of court if there is a failure to comply with the order. Before providing the information, practitioners should wait for a court order or a subpoena to appear as a witness or provide the information. Where the order or subpoena is by a tribunal, it may be advisable for a practitioner to ensure that the statutory powers of the tribunal allow the enforcement of the tendering of the information sought. If a lawyer acting for a client requests a copy of records without a court order, and if the practitioner chooses to supply them, a cautious approach would be to seek express consent for that release from the client.
* *If there is a serious, identifiable risk to a third party.* Where there is a serious, fore-seeable risk to an identified third party (for example, a client reveals their intent to physically harm or kill another person), one US authority[75] suggests that this might justify revealing confidential information. It is not possible to confidently predict whether this decision is applicable in Australia because no court here has applied it. If it is intended to rely on this decision, disclosure should only be made to those persons who need to be advised—that is, the target of the threat and/or the police.
* *Public interest.* The English authority of *W v Egdell*[76] suggested that in some cir-cumstances confidential information can be revealed where it is in the public interest. In that case, a psychiatrist was concerned about the violent tendencies of a client. The psychiatrist revealed the content of a report, made after consul-tation with the client, to a tribunal reviewing that client's case. The judgement supported that breach of confidence as there was a real risk of danger to the public rather than mere speculation or risk. It would be very rare for this sort of situa-tion to arise for a complementary medicine practitioner. To date, there is no clear authority suggesting that this would be a reason for disclosure of the confidential information in Australia.

Remedies for breach of confidence

Should a breach of confidence occur, the remedies available to a client potentially would be to:

* sue for breach of confidence
* seek an injunction to stop a breach of the obligation

- seek recovery in negligence for any damage that may be suffered
- sue in contract for a breach of the implied term
- sue in defamation, or
- commence professional misconduct proceedings.

Privacy Act

The *Privacy Act 1988* (Cth) ('Privacy Act') impacts upon the practice of private health services providers such as medical doctors, private hospitals, nurses and many other health services providers such as complementary medicine practitioners, including but not limited to herbalists, naturopaths, massage therapists, traditional Chinese medicine practitioners, chiropractors and osteopaths. As this list is not exhaustive, it is safe to assume that all complementary medicine practitioners are subject to this statute. The provisions of the *Health Records Act 2001* (Vic), the *Health Records Information Privacy Act 2002* (NSW) and the *Health Records (Privacy and Access) Act 1997* (ACT) incorporate similar but not identical principles. It is not possible to deal with every provision in this legislation but this treatment provides a broad overview of important considerations. Currently the *Privacy Act* is relevant to all private health services providers anywhere in Australia. 'NSW, Victoria and the Australian Capital Territory private sector health service providers must comply with both Australian and state or territory privacy laws when handling health information.'[77]

The current legislative arrangements are an amalgam of Commonwealth and state provisions that creates some difficulty in appreciating which provisions apply to a specific circumstance. The Office of the Australian Information Commissioner has published the *Guide to Health Privacy* (Guidelines) which provides an overview of the obligations for health service providers including the *Privacy Act* and the Australian Privacy Principles (APP).[78]

To what information does the legislation apply?

The *Privacy Act* applies to 'personal information' (PI)—that is, information about a natural person who can be identified from that information. The *Privacy Act* also regulates the use of 'health information', which is a subset of personal information. Health information is 'sensitive information' that has some stricter requirements and includes matters:

- about a person's individual health or disability at any time
- about expressed wishes regarding future health services
- about health services provided to a person, and
- collected while providing the health service.

Health information can include medical information, name, address, Medicare number, and notes or opinions about a person's health status. It would include matters such as information about a person's physical or mental health, prescriptions or test results.

The Office of the Australian Information Commissioner has developed thirteen legally binding Australian Privacy Principles (APP) and the Guidelines to explain how these principles should be applied. Although not legally binding, the Guidelines are intended to assist health professionals to comply with this legislation.

This treatment does not deal with all the relevant privacy issues that arise for health practices but it provides a selection of significant requirements focussed primarily on matters that may be most significant for complementary medicine practitioners.

Chapter 1: Key steps to embedding privacy in your health practice[79]

The Guidelines seek to meet privacy obligations the practical steps of which should be:

Step 1 *Develop and implement a privacy management plan* (PMP)—A PMP suggests four steps to incorporate a 'culture of privacy'; 'robust and effective privacy processes'; evaluation of the processes to ensure effectiveness and enhancing responses based upon privacy issues that arise.[80] The intention is that the PMP will demonstrate the alignment of the practice business with policy obligations.[81]

Step 2 *Develop clear lines of accountability for privacy management*—which would include clarity about which staff have the expertise and responsibility for privacy issues or provide for designated privacy officers in larger healthcare practices to deal with questions or incidents that may arise.

Step 3 *Create a documented record of the types of personal information you handle*—which requires understanding of the holdings of personal information such as client clinical records; general client issues such as contact information and medicare details or specialist reports, how personal information is received and where is it held such as electronic records; at the clinic or off site and cloud storage.

Step 4 *Understand your privacy obligations*—and implement processes such as addressing the handling information from collection to use and disclosure to storage, security and when information is no longer required; provide the means for clients to access and correct personal information and process for receiving and responding to privacy enquiries and complaints.[82]

Step 5 *Staff training*—which would involve training of new staff; having good processes for staff to understand their obligations; holding information sessions and facilitation of professional development opportunities in this area.

Step 6 *Create an APP privacy policy*—which deals with kinds of PI collected and held; how to collect and hold PI; the purposes to collect, hold, use and disclose personal information; the means to access to PI and seek correction; and complaints process.

Step 7 *Take reasonable steps to protect and secure personal information*—which would 'protect the personal information you hold from misuse, interference, loss, and from unauthorised access, modification or disclosure, destroy or de-identify personal information you hold once it is no longer needed.'[83]

Chapter 2: Collecting health information

Health information can be collected if 'the patient consents (expressly or impliedly) to you collecting it, and the information is reasonably necessary for your activities (which would generally be providing a health service to that patient)'.[84] An obvious example would be when a client described to a health practitioner the symptoms that would be an example of a collection that would be reasonably necessary for the activity.

The health information should only be collected by the client directly with the practitioner 'unless it is not reasonable to practical to do so'.[85] Examples of circumstances where collecting health information directly from a patient may not be reasonable or practicable would be an emergency or where a client is a child or a person without capacity which may require a parent or guardian. It should be understood that when collecting health information in an area such as a waiting room, provision should be made for a private room or music that prevents sensitive information being passed in the waiting room.

Privacy notices—when collecting health information a client must be informed of why the information is collected and how that information will be handled.[86]

This information should be provided before the collection or soon after the collection. The Guidelines suggest the privacy notice should include:

- details of the person collecting the health information and contact details
- 'whether the collection is required or authorised by law
- the purposes of collection
- any consequences for the patient if the health information is not collected
- that your Australian Privacy Principles (APP) privacy policy contains information on:
- how patients can access and correct the health information you hold about them
- how patients can make a complaint about how you handle their health information, and details of how you will deal with a complaint
- whether you are likely to disclose health information overseas (and if so, where)'.[87]

Notice might be provided by notice in the waiting room or leaflet with the required information or the details of collection on a paper or online form or orally, but a written notice may be best to ensure the required details are covered.

The *Privacy Act* requires a health practitioner to consider if it is possible to give clients the option of not identifying themselves or using a pseudonym. This is possible, but a health practitioner does not have to deal with a person who is anonymous or pseudonymous if the health practitioner is required by law or a court or tribunal to deal with persons who have identified themselves, or if it is not practical to deal with a person who is anonymous or pseudonymous.[88]

Chapter 3: Using or disclosing health information

A health practitioner can use or disclose health information 'for the primary purpose for which it was collected or for a secondary purpose in certain circumstances'.[89] A primary purpose is the main activity for which the health information is collected. In a normal clinical situation the health information is used to provide the services to diagnose and treat the client. The focus is to ensure that the use of health information is in a manner that the client would expect and they would not be surprised by its use.[90]

A purpose other than a primary purpose will be a secondary purpose. A secondary purpose can be applied if the client has given consent. In addition, a secondary purpose can be applied if the use was reasonably expected and it is for a purpose that is directly related to the primary purpose of the collection. This determination relies upon the community expectation of how information would be applied and the nature of the information provided by the health practitioner.[91]

Examples of an appropriate use of a secondary purpose would be where a practitioner refers the patient to another practitioner such as a GP or another complementary medicine practitioner, or where there is a multi-disciplinary team when the client has been made aware of the nature of the practice and the possibility of other members of the team accessing the health information. A different position would apply if the client has indicated that the team based approach was not acceptable to them.[92] Other examples would be billing; management, quality assurance; disclosure to an expert for a medico-legal opinion, an insurer, or a Medicare audit.

There is also some leeway to use or disclose health information where it is unreasonable or impracticable to obtain consent to the use or disclosure, and you reasonably believe the use or disclosure is necessary to lessen or prevent a serious threat to the life, health or safety of any individual, or to public health or safety.[93]

Chapter 4: Giving access to health information

Clients are entitled to access information held by the practitioner, with that access required within 30 calendar days unless an exception applies or if access is unreasonable or impracticable. In the circumstances that a health practitioner refuses to give access to the health information or refuses to provide access in the manner sought by the client, the health practitioner should take reasonable steps to deal with the access that suits both the practitioner and the client and provide a written notice setting out the grounds of the refusal and the mechanism for complaint.[94] Chapter 4 page 2 of the Guidelines provides a flow chart of the access requirements which is useful.

For obvious reasons it is important to ensure the request for access is made by the client or some other authorised person, particularly when the client is not well known.[95] The Guidelines set out some grounds for refusing access which include:

- the health practitioner reasonably believes access would pose a serious threat to the life, health or safety of any individual or to public health or public safety[96]
- the request is frivolous or vexatious
- it involves information relevant to legal proceedings between the practitioner and client or it would reveal intentions in relation to negotiations between the practitioner and client or would reveal evaluative information that is part of the commercially sensitive decision-making process of the health practitioner.
- to provide access would be unlawful or not permitting access is required by law
- the practitioner has reason to suspect illegal activity or serious misconduct related to the work of the practitioner or providing access may prejudice activities of an enforcement body.

Further significant matters for consideration[97]

Access to health information can be provided:

- electronically or by hard copy
- allowing the client to view the information
- providing information by phone
- providing an accurate summary
- providing a video or audio recording

A practitioner should comply with the type of access sought unless it is unreasonable or impracticable to do so. It is possible to charge for providing access as long as it is not excessive.

Chapter 5: Correcting health information

Reasonable steps should be taken to ensure the health information held by the practitioner is correct whether there is a request to correct information or you become aware that the practitioner holds incorrect health information. Incorrect information would be where there is an error or the information is out of date, incomplete, irrelevant or misleading.[98]

Chapter 6: Health management activities

The Guidelines suggest that 'Provided certain requirements are met, you can collect health information where it is necessary for health management activities. You can use or disclose health information for health management activities in accordance with the usual use and disclosure principles.'[99]

   This relates to normal activities for the running of the health service, such as quality assurance or where a health insurer seeks to collect information relevant to a possible fraud. This type of collection can occur without consent where it is necessary for health management activities and cannot be done with de-identified information, it is impracticable to obtain consent and is required under an Australian law.[100]

Chapter 7: Disclosing information about patients with impaired capacity

In the case of a dealing with a person with impaired capacity it is possible to disclose a patient's health information to a 'responsible person' where:[101]

*   'the patient lacks the capacity to consent or is unable to communicate consent, and
*   the disclosure is either necessary to provide appropriate treatment, or is made for compassionate reasons'.

Chapter 8: Using and disclosing genetic information in the case of a serious threat

There is room to allow use or disclosure of genetic information in specific circumstances. The Guidelines suggest:

> Provided certain conditions are met, you can use or disclose a patient's genetic information without consent where you reasonably believe the use or disclosure is necessary to lessen or prevent a serious threat to the life health or safety of a genetic relative of the patient.[102]

This would require reference to Australian Privacy Principles guidelines that are issued by the National Health and Medical Research Council under s 95AA of the *Privacy Act*.

Chapter 9: Research

The Guidelines suggest:

> Provided certain requirements are met you can collect health information where it is necessary for research, or the compilation or analysis of statistics, relevant to

public health or public safety you can use or disclose health information where it is necessary for research, or the compilation or analysis of statistics, relevant to public health or public safety.[103]

Normally consent is required for the use of health information but it is possible to collect health information without consent when:

- it is necessary for research, or compiling statistics relevant to public health or public safety and
- where the research cannot be done using de-identified information
- it is impracticable to obtain consent and
- it is required by Australian law (not the Privacy Act) or complies with other regulations and expectations for these actions.[104]

In New Zealand, the *Privacy Act 1993* applies similar principles in relation to an agency (any person or body of person corporate or incorporate in the public or private sector) collecting personal information about an identifiable person.

General medical practitioners

A practitioner may consider it important that a client maintain contact with their general medical practitioner. A client may not share this desire for various reasons. As disclosure of confidential information to a general medical practitioner may breach confidence, express consent from the client should be obtained.[105]

Notifiable diseases

There may be some clinical advantages to identifying cases of diseases such as venereal disease, tuberculosis and poliomyelitis that medical practitioners and other health practitioners may be obliged to report to relevant state authorities. Complementary medicine practitioners have no legal obligation to notify any authority. If the practitioner thinks a client has a notifiable disease, they should strongly encourage the client to seek medical attention.

Child abuse reporting

Voluntary reporting

In most Australian jurisdictions, and in New Zealand,[106] any person may report to authorities that a child or young person is being maltreated or is in need of care. The relevant statutes normally provide statutory protection to a person who acts reasonably in making that report.

Mandatory reporting

In the jurisdictions specified below, health professionals such as medical doctors, nurses, social workers and in some contexts complementary medicine practitioners are obliged to report suspected child abuse to the relevant authorities.[107]

The Northern Territory has very significant provisions in this area that impact on ordinary citizens and registered health practitioners. Section 26 of the *Care and Protection of Children Act* (NT) states that a person is guilty of an offence if the person believes, on reasonable grounds, that a child has suffered or is likely to suffer harm or exploitation; a child aged less than fourteen years has been or is likely to be a victim of a sexual offence; or a child has been or is likely to be a victim of an offence against section 128 of the Criminal Code; and does not, as soon as possible after forming that belief, report (orally or in writing) to the CEO of the department administering the legislation or a police officer. A registered health practitioner may be liable under section 26 if they believe, on reasonable grounds, that a child aged at least fourteen years (but less than sixteen years) has been or is likely to be a victim of a sexual offence; and that the difference in age between the child and alleged sexual offender is more than two years; and does not report this to the CEO or a police officer.

In New South Wales, section 27 of the *Children and Young Persons (Care and Protection) Act 1998* applies to a person who, in the course of his or her professional work or other paid employment, or in a management position for an organisation, delivers health care, welfare, education, children's services, residential services or law enforcement, wholly or partly, to children. If a person to whom this section applies has reasonable grounds to suspect that a child is at risk of significant harm, the person has a duty to report it. This provision might in some cases involve a complementary medicine practitioner. Section 29 provides protection from legal action to a person who makes a report in good faith. Similar provisions in South Australia are found in sections 30 and 31 of the *Children and Young People (Safety) Act 2017* (SA).

Section 28 of the *Children, Youth and Families Act 2005* (Vic) states that a person may make a report to the secretary if the person has a significant concern for the well-being of a child. The provisions of sections 182–189 of the *Children, Youth and Families Act 2005* (Vic) require a report to be made about child abuse if the person concerned has a post-secondary qualification in youth, social or welfare work and works in health, education or community welfare services. This provision might include a complementary medicine practitioner with the relevant qualification.

Client records

To properly service your client, to inform colleagues and employees treating that client and for professional indemnity insurance purposes, it is important to keep proper records of consultations, treatments and advice. Client records comprise files, notes of treatment, prescriptions, medical history, personal details, letters to other practitioners, test results, x-rays, diagnosis, family history, photographs and correspondence with clients.

Purpose of records

Maintaining good records is an important feature of competent professional practice. Good records contain important information such as warnings or consents given, details such as allergies to drugs or substances, referrals made, treatment and advice given, and progress made by the client. Another practitioner may rely on these records in treating the client, and their clarity and completeness may be vital.

BOX 3.4

Practice tip

Should liability or ethical issues arise, an established habit of maintaining thorough and correct records will add weight to the evidence of a practitioner who states that a specific answer, question, warning or advice was or was not given.

Client access to records

A client may seek access to records for a number of reasons:

- to assist in treatment by another practitioner
- to correct errors
- to provide the basis for an action or complaint against the practitioner or another practitioner, and
- to check the information provided to the practitioner by third parties such as other practitioners or family members.

Some practitioners may happily provide access to these records and/or provide copies. Others may have concerns about such access because:

- the records may contain potentially defamatory comments
- the client will not understand them, or
- the client will find the records confusing.

The provisions of the *Privacy Act* (discussed above, pages 52–57) now specify that a client is entitled to access their records, to obtain a copy, and to correct and update these records.

BOX 3.5

Practice tips: Keeping records

Client records may be read by persons other than the practitioner, such as a client or other party in the context of litigation. Client records should[108]

- be legible and in English
- be concise, accurate and complete
- not contain value judgements and conclusions
- contain only readily understood abbreviations, and
- avoid any comments that could be embarrassing for the practitioner or client.

Practice tip: Letter of confirmation

A letter or email of confirmation to the client of advice or warnings given provides excellent evidence for a practitioner and is difficult to deny as evidence. This is an important measure when the practitioner thinks that significant oral advice has been given to a client and it is important to confirm both that this conversation has occurred and been understood such as the need to provide a specific dose of herbs or other ingestive substances or the details of an eating program. That is advisable for the benefit of the client and practitioner. Contemporaneous file notes are helpful and necessary, but a timely letter or email can confirm what has passed between a client and a practitioner in the case of a difference in evidence between client and practitioner at a later date. It is important to keep a copy of that letter or email and, in the case of an email, obtain acknowledgement of receipt.

BOX 3.6

Practice tip: Do's and don'ts of keeping practice records

- Keep individual health records. Keep a readily accessible individual health record for each client, even if other family members are also being treated.
- Be accurate. The accuracy of records kept may be an important factor in litigation. For example, if a practitioner states that he or she performed some professional service on a specified date and the plaintiff can establish that he or she was interstate on that date, this may undermine the perceived reliability of that person's evidence. A small inaccuracy in record-keeping may cast doubt on the thoroughness of the records and the professionalism of the practitioner. Where the practitioner and client disagree about what was said and done, the accuracy and thoroughness of the practitioner's records may be vital.
- Use a client sign-in sheet. A client sign-in sheet can verify the date a client visited a clinic for treatment. This can confirm inconsistencies in the evidence of a client should litigation ensue.
- Keep records of the subjective responses of the client. A client may complain that they have derived little or no benefit from treatment. Practitioners should record any improvement or worsening of the client's condition on the client record. Subjective reports, recorded as they happened by the client, will carry more weight than the notes of the practitioner and will be difficult to rebut as evidence. A client progress form can indicate progress or regression as the treatment regime continues at various intervals. If a plateau is reached in the therapeutic process, this information can be revisited to confirm to the client the benefits felt earlier in the process.
- Maintain up-to-date records. Records will provide the maximum protection for a practitioner if they are an on-the-spot, honest and accurate account of what took place.
- Properly identify the record. The record should reveal the relevant date and time, in chronological and logical order.
- Record client non-compliance. This may have a bearing on contributory negligence and the general impression of the client in litigation. The term 'DNKA' (did not keep appointment) can be used for non-attendance at an appointment. Notes can incorporate failure to do exercises or to adopt lifestyle changes, and avoidance of specific activities such as lifting.
- Keep records indefinitely. Injury may not become obvious until some time after treatment, so records should be kept indefinitely.
- Fill in all blanks on forms. If blanks are left in a form, this might suggest an error, oversight or lack of thoroughness.
- Don't erase. If an amendment is necessary, cross through the entry, insert the correction, and sign and date the amendment. This is less likely to be seen as a

fraudulent entry because there is no attempt to conceal the correction. An entry erasure will raise suspicion that it was altered at a later date to support the practitioner's claim. Hard copy records should be kept in pen. Records kept in pencil will invite questions about whether the record was altered subsequently.

- Don't skip lines or leave spaces. This may suggest that the space was left for insertion of further information. It is particularly suspicious if an important entry has been placed in a position that normally would have been left as space.
- Don't squeeze in notes. This will suggest subsequent tampering, even if it was a genuine entry done at the time.
- Don't use words such as 'routine' or 'inadvertent'. The use of the word 'routine' to indicate a normal or standard situation in regard to treatment may be viewed as indicating a lack of consideration of the specific case at hand or a matter not demanding attention. The term 'inadvertent', when referring to an accidental or unexpected result, may be interpreted as meaning inattentive or heedless. Refer also to Clause 8.4, 'Health Records', AHPRA Code of Conduct 2022 (https://www.chinesemedicineboard.gov.au/Codes-Guidelines/Code-of-conduct.aspx).

Practice tip: Test your records

To test whether your records are sufficiently comprehensive to withstand the litigation process, take a number of old files from previous years and answer the following questions:

BOX 3.7

Testing your practice records

- On a specific date, was the client's condition improving or had it worsened?
- Did the client make any statements as to their condition?
- What treatment was given?

If you are unable to answer these questions, perhaps you are not keeping sufficiently complete records[109]

Case study

A South Australian District Court case, *Edwards v Butler*,[110] emphasises the importance of good clinical records. Here a therapeutic massage therapist was subject to a claim for breach of contract and negligence over what the client alleged was a neck manipulation that caused personal injury. The practitioner denied that the manipulation had occurred.

The pivotal issue was whether the client's or practitioner's version of events was to be accepted. The practitioner did not have any recollection of the treatment provided on the relevant date or record, and he relied substantially upon what was his 'practice' to determine what had happened. The defendant stated that his clients would normally fill out an information sheet, but it appears that this was not available for the court. In the absence of satisfactory evidence to support the defendant's version of events, the judge accepted the evidence of the client, whom the judge considered to be a most impressive witness. Judgement was made in favour of the client/plaintiff in that case.

Disciplinary action

The professional association's code of ethics provisions should provide details of why and how action may be brought against a practitioner for alleged professional misconduct. Practitioners are entitled to a reasonable opportunity to defend any claim made against them, as an adverse finding may have important professional, social and economic consequences. Practitioners should not ignore any action taken against them because a decision may be made in their absence. It is much more difficult to overturn a decision than to defend the decision in the first instance.

Generally, any disciplinary proceedings should exhibit the following features:

- reasonable notice in writing of the venue date and time of any hearing
- sufficient details of the charge made to allow the practitioner to prepare a case to answer the charge
- an opportunity to be heard before a body that is not biased, and
- the tribunal conforming to the relevant disciplinary provisions.

General comments

The disciplinary provisions of some codes of ethics are substantial and complex, while others are very basic. Disciplinary proceedings against a practitioner can seriously affect his or her professional reputation, as they may lead to expulsion from the organisation, suspension, fines or other penalties. Expulsion or suspension will deny access to the advantages of membership, including the perception of quality that membership may provide. These potentially serious consequences entitle a practitioner to expect a reasonable level of sophistication and fairness in the disciplinary process.

Need for provision for sanctions

Some codes of ethics specify ethical practices but don't contain disciplinary provisions. Unless the rules of the association permit expulsion or other sanction, there is no power to discipline a practitioner for a breach of the code of ethics.

Vague provisions

Some codes of ethics give little detail other than a reference to a disciplinary committee. Vague disciplinary provisions give practitioners little guidance as to their entitlements and the possible consequences of a breach of professional rules. This does not assist in the development of ethical practices within the profession. A lack of detail may mean that appropriate procedures will be implied by a court if there is a requirement to review the decision-making process.

Jurisdiction of the courts

Disciplinary action may affect the ability of a person to earn an income. For this reason, if requested, a court may have jurisdiction to consider whether the proceedings were conducted fairly.

Misconduct in registered professions

Under the National Law, there is provision for notifications to be made to a national board of a registered profession in relation to alleged misconduct of a registered health practitioner. A national board may decide not to refer the matter to a responsible tribunal, which is the local tribunal given jurisdiction to deal with misconduct matters in each jurisdiction. A national board may choose to caution the health practitioner or apply conditions to their practice.[111] A national board may constitute a health panel if the board thinks the practitioner may have an impairment. If a national board considers that, based on a notification or for any other reason, the practitioner may have behaved in a way that constitutes 'unsatisfactory professional performance' or 'unprofessional conduct', it may constitute a performance and professional standards panel to consider the matter. In a case of more serious misconduct where 'professional misconduct' may have occurred or the registration was improperly obtained, the matter must be referred to the responsible tribunal. This step may be requested by the practitioner. A performance and professional standards panel must refer a matter to the tribunal if it considers that a matter before it could constitute professional misconduct.

Professional misconduct is defined in section 5 of the National Law to include:

- unprofessional conduct by the practitioner that amounts to conduct that is substantially below the standard reasonably expected of a registered health practitioner of an equivalent level of training or experience, and
- more than one instance of unprofessional conduct that, when considered together, amounts to conduct that is substantially below the standard reasonably expected of a registered health practitioner of an equivalent level of training or experience, and
- conduct of the practitioner, whether occurring in connection with the practice of the health practitioner's profession or not, that is inconsistent with the practitioner being a fit and proper person to hold registration in the profession.

Provision is usually made for various types of orders by the responsible tribunal, including:

- caution or reprimand
- orders for further education, training or counselling
- a period of supervised practice or limits on practice
- fines
- suspension (only available for a tribunal), and
- cancellation of registration (only available for a tribunal).

Generally, the provisions require a practitioner to be given notice of the proceedings and of the charges made. Where deregistration is possible, the practitioner will usually have an entitlement to seek to be represented by a lawyer and will enjoy a right of appeal to a court or tribunal in some cases.

The common law requires tribunals and bodies charged with the role of adjudicating on the registration status of practitioners to apply procedural fairness unless the statute specifically excludes this requirement. A court will be slow to exclude the obligation to observe procedural fairness unless this is specified clearly in the legislation.[112]

Procedural fairness (sometimes called natural justice) requires an individual to be afforded the opportunity to be heard and to present their case before a tribunal or another body that makes a decision that will affect the person's rights or entitlements. Additionally, the body making the decision should not be perceived as biased or prejudiced. The requirement for procedural fairness will vary, depending on the particular circumstances of a case.[113]

Mandatory notifications under the National Law

One significant ethical issue that will arise under the National Law is the compulsory requirement for registered health practitioners, employers and educational providers to notify the National Agency as soon as practicable if they form a reasonable belief that another registered health practitioner has behaved in a way that constitutes notifiable conduct or a student has an impairment that may place the public at substantial risk of harm. Notifiable conduct is defined in section 140 as:

- practising while intoxicated by drugs or alcohol
- engaging in sexual misconduct in connection with professional practice
- placing the public at risk of substantial harm as the practitioner is impaired, or
- placing the public at risk of harm by a significant departure from accepted professional standards.

A failure to make that notification is not an offence but may be subject to action. Note that there are some exceptions which may apply to the obligation to notify under section 141(4) of the National Law. An employer has the same obligation to notify the National Agency of notifiable conduct by an employee under section 142.

An education provider must notify the National Agency if the provider reasonably believes a student has an impairment that may place the public at substantial risk of harm.

Not surprisingly, there is provision in section 237 of the National Law for protection from civil or criminal liability or under an administrative process for a person making a notification in good faith. In addition, the making of a notification or giving information is not a breach of professional etiquette or ethics, or a departure from accepted standards of professional conduct. Refer to the AHPRA Guidelines for Mandatory Notifications about registered health practitioners (March 2020), which provide more detail.[114]

Obligations of disciplinary tribunals and committees

The discussion in this section will focus on the principles that might apply to hearings by professional bodies for non-registered professions. An example would be a charge of professional misconduct against a naturopath or homoeopath heard by a disciplinary committee in accordance with the rules of a professional association.

Jurisdiction of the courts

A court may overturn a decision of a disciplinary committee. This might occur if the hearing does not provide the appropriate level of procedural fairness or if there is a failure to comply with any specified rules for the hearing. A court will be slow to intervene in the internal affairs of a professional body unless it can be shown that such an intervention is necessary to avoid unfair practice.[115]

If an intervention does occur, the court will not re-hear the case. Rather, the court will review the procedures taken and decision made to ascertain whether this justifies the decision being set aside.[116] A court will ascertain whether the decision had some basis or evidence to support it, even if it was a decision that the court would not have reached.

A court will only intervene if it is legally justified, such as where the disciplinary act is a restraint of trade. The restraint of trade basis for intervention might arise where the disciplinary proceedings could stop or restrict the ability of a practitioner to practise his or her profession. Examples of situations where a court might overturn a decision are where:

- the penalty applied is disproportionate to the offence—that is, expulsion is ordered where a fine or reprimand would have been sufficient—or
- there was a lack of procedural fairness.

Important considerations in disciplinary proceedings

This discussion must be general because the rules of each professional body are different and the circumstances of each case are unique. Observance of these procedural issues will limit the likelihood of a successful court challenge and, importantly, provide the basis of fairer and more open proceedings.

- *Observance of specified procedures.* The provisions that describe disciplinary proceedings should be followed closely. The non-observance of prescribed procedures may be the basis for a court to set aside a decision. Only those officers duly appointed for that purpose by the relevant rules should conduct disciplinary proceedings. Outsiders to the body should not be involved unless the rules permit.[117]
- *Express power to expel.* A member of a voluntary association can only be expelled or disciplined if there is an express power to do so. Such a power is not implied.[118]
- *Properly constituted body.* The body hearing the disciplinary matter should be properly constituted. All committee members eligible for the hearing should be properly notified to avoid a perception of stacking.[119] Any specified majority for a decision—that is, a special or simple majority—should be observed.
- *Definition of misconduct.* The rules do not need to specify detailed criteria for what constitutes misconduct if the general ground of misconduct is provided for and is rationally applied.
- *Procedural fairness.* A common reason for setting aside a decision is the failure to observe procedural fairness.[120] A court will usually imply this obligation even if there is nothing stated in the rules.
- *Notice.* An important aspect of procedural fairness is the need to give proper notice. The requirements of proper notice are:
  - It must include details of the charge being brought against the practitioner, including the stipulation said to have been breached, the factual circumstances and details of the person who has made the complaint.

- It should list the issues likely to be canvassed in the hearing.
- It should specify the place, date and time at which the hearing will be held. The notice should give sufficient time for the practitioner charged to make inquiries, to consider their position and to formulate responses.[121] The appropriate length of notice will depend on matters such as the express provisions of the rules, and the complexity and seriousness of the charges. In this, it is best to err on the side of generosity. If there is doubt about whether sufficient time has been given, the practitioner charged should be asked whether they require further time for preparation.
- The notice can be oral, but prudence would suggest it should always be in writing.
- It should indicate possible outcomes of the meeting if the charge is proved—that is, fine, reprimand, suspension or expulsion—and the consequences if the practitioner does not appear at the hearing.

- *Non-appearance at hearing.* Procedural fairness is designed to provide a person with an opportunity to be heard.[122] If a party has been given proper notice and they don't appear, the matter can proceed in their absence. If a good excuse for non-appearance is provided, a re-hearing should be scheduled.[123]
- *Legal representation.* There is normally no entitlement to legal representation unless the rules provide otherwise, especially when there is an appeal to another body where representation is permitted. The law is somewhat uncertain on this point.[124]
- *Onus of proof.* The onus to prove the charge is on the body that hears the matter. The practitioner is not obliged to prove their innocence.
- *Standard of proof.* The standard of proof (that is, the level of proof to which the charge needs to be proven) is usually described as higher than the civil standard of proof ('on the balance of probabilities') but not as high as the criminal law standard of proof ('beyond reasonable doubt').
- *Rules of evidence.* In formal court proceedings, the common law and statutes apply a complex set of rules of evidence, which indicate what is or is not admissible evidence in court. These rules often substantially limit access to certain types of evidence. These rules do not apply to these tribunals. Despite this, a tribunal should not rely heavily on hearsay evidence—that is, evidence from a person who heard what someone else said, without any independent understanding of the facts.
- *Appeal right.* Procedural fairness can be satisfied without an entitlement to appeal to another internal body.[125]
- *Reasons for decision.* A judge in a court of law will always provide reasons for a decision. There have been different views expressed about the obligation to provide reasons in the context of bodies such as disciplinary committees. The preponderance of authority suggests that there is no obligation to provide reasons for a decision, although the status of a decision may be enhanced by publishing reasons.
- Publishing reasons may, however, provide fertile ground for appeal. The reasons given may indicate that the decision was based on irrelevant, erroneous or improper grounds. The absence of reasons may in some contexts suggest that there were no good reasons for the decision.[126]

BOX 3.8

Practice tip: Reasons for decisions

If it is intended to provide reasons, Forbes[127] has suggested some guidelines that might be followed:

- State the charge or issue for decision. For example: 'The charge is that practitioner James Knight has breached rule 15 of the code of ethics in that he has claimed personally and in advertisement a qualification as a sports medicine massage therapist without actually having that qualification.'
- Recite the rule or provision that governs the issue or charge. 'Rule 15 states ...'
- If there is some dispute as to the interpretation of the rule, state the preferred interpretation. 'The rule provides that a practitioner must not make any representation of a qualification that is false or misleading. The practitioner argued that this referred to representation in advertising only. The committee interprets this provision to mean representation whether in person, orally, in writing or on a sign or advertisement.'
- Summarise the relevant evidence, pointing out important matters of dispute, corroboration (which is the confirmation of one piece of evidence by another source) and the version of the evidence that is preferred.
- If inferences are drawn from circumstantial evidence, make a decision on these facts and then indicate the inference drawn.
- Apply the governing rule to the facts and inferences found.
- State clearly the decision and any orders that might be needed to implement that decision.

Notes

1 M. Coady & S. Bloch, *Codes of Ethics and the Professions*, Melbourne University Press, Melbourne, 1996, p. 15.
2 M.-J. Johnstone, *Bioethics—A Nursing Perspective*, 5th ed., Churchill Livingstone, Sydney, 2009, p. 12.
3 W.T. Reich, Introduction to the *Encyclopaedia of Bioethics*, revised ed., Simon & Schuster Macmillan, New York, 1995, p. xxi from Johnstone, *Bioethics—A Nursing Perspective*, p. 13.
4 Ibid., p. 14.
5 K. Danner Clouser et al., 'Informed Consent and Alternative Medicine' (1996) 2 *Alternative Therapies* 76.
6 Stone & Matthews, *Complementary Medicine and the Law*, Oxford University Press, 1996, p. 233.
7 T.L. Beauchamp & J.F. Childress, *Principles of Biomedical Ethics,* 5th ed., Oxford University Press, New York, 2001, p. 3.
8 B. Richards & J. Louise, *Medical Law and Ethics: A Problem-Based Approach,* Lexis Nexis Butterworths, Sydney, 2014, p. 7.
9 Stone & Matthews, *Complementary Medicine and the Law*, Oxford University Press, 1996, p. 235.
10 J.F. Allen, *Health Law and Medical Ethics for Health Professionals*, Pearson, Boston, 2013, p. 144.
11 Richards & Louise, *Medical Law and Ethics*, Lexis Nexis Butterworths, 2014, p. 9.
12 Johnstone, *Bioethics—A Nursing Perspective*, 5th ed., Churchill Livingstone, Sydney, 2009, p. 23

13 Ibid., p. 73.
14 P.Y. Windt et al., *Ethical Issues in the Professions*, Prentice-Hall, Englewood Cliffs, NJ, 1989, p. 99.
15 Coady & Bloch, *Codes of Ethics and the Professions*, p. 73.
16 Beauchamp & Childress, *Principles of Biomedical Ethics*, p. 12.
17 Richards & Louise, *Medical Law and Ethics*, p. 11.
18 Stone & Matthews, *Complementary Medicine and the Law*, Chapter 13, p. 19.
19 Ibid., p. 235.
20 J. Devereux, *Australian Medical Law*, 3rd ed., Routledge-Cavendish, Abingdon, 2007, p. 6.
21 Stone & Matthews, *Complementary Medicine and the Law*, p. 238; J. Stone, *An Ethical Framework for Complementary and Alternative Therapies*, Routledge, New York, 2002, pp. viii, 3, 13.
22 E. Ernst, 'The Ethics of Complementary Medicine' (1996) 22 *Journal of Medical Ethics* 197 at 198.
23 N. Lynoe, 'Ethical Professional Aspects of the Practice of Alternative Medicine' (1992) 20 *Scandinavian Journal of Social Medicine* 217.
24 Stone, *An Ethical Framework*, p. 34.
25 S. Fulder, *The Handbook of Alternative and Complementary Medicine*, 3rd ed., Oxford University Press, New York, 1996, p. 6.
26 Beauchamp & Childress, *Principles of Biomedical Ethics*, p. 99; Stone & Matthews, *Complementary Medicine and the Law*, p. 257.
27 B.B. O'Connor, *Healing Traditions: Alternative Medicine and the Health Professions*, University of Pennsylvania Press, Philadelphia, PA, 1995, p. 181.
28 Reflected in the High Court decision of *Rogers v Whitaker* (1992) 109 ALR 625 at 628.
29 Johnstone, *Bioethics—A Nursing Perspective*, p. 45.
30 Article 25 (10 December 1948).
31 Johnstone, *Bioethics—A Nursing Perspective*, p. 138.
32 House of Lords Science and Technology Committee, *Sixth Report Session 1999–2000*: Complementary and Alternative Medicine, Select Committee Report, Her Majesty's Government, London, 2000, para. 4.7; Ernst, 'The Ethics of Complementary Medicine', p. 199.
33 M.H. Kottow, 'Classical Medicine v Alternative Medical Practices', (1992) 18 *Journal of Medical Ethics* 18 at 21.
34 J. Sugarman & L. Burk, 'Physicians' Ethical Obligations Regarding Alternative Medicine' (1998) 280 *Journal of American Medical Association* 1623 at 1625.
35 Stone & Matthews, *Complementary Medicine and the Law*, p. 268.
36 New Zealand government (NZ Report), *Chiropractic in New Zealand: Report of the Commission of Inquiry*, New Zealand Government, Wellington, 1979, pp. 30–1. 34.
37 For example, the Therapeutic Goods Administration 'Guidelines on the Evidence Required to Support Indications for other Listable Medicines', 2014.
38 H.S. Berliner, 'Scientific Medicine Since Flexner', in W. Salmon (ed.), *Alternative Medicines: Popular and Policy Perspectives*, Tavistock, London, 1984, p. 47.
39 A point not readily acknowledged by many OM writers: L.J. Schneiderman, 'Medical Ethics and Alternative Medicine' (1998) 2 *Scientific Review of Alternative Medicine* 63; John S Garrow, 'How Much of Orthodox Medicine is Evidence Based?' (2007) 335 *British Medical Journal*, 951.
40 H. Brody et al., 'Ethics at the Interface of Conventional and Complementary Medicine', in W.B. Jonas & J.S. Levin (eds), *Essentials of Complementary and Alternative Medicine*, Lippincott Williams and Wilkins, Baltimore, MD, 1999, p. 52.
41 House of Lords Science and Technology Committee, *Sixth Report Session 1999–2000* para. 14.20.
42 Sugarman & Burk, 'Physicians' Ethical Obligations', at 1623, 1625.
43 J.F. Drane (ed.), *Encyclopedia of Bioethics*, Macmillan, New York, 1997, p. 141.
44 House of Lords Science and Technology Committee, *Sixth Report Session 1999–2000*, para. 3.3.
45 Sugarman & Burk, 'Physicians' Ethical Obligations', at 1623.

46 N. Lynoe, 'Ethical Professional Aspects', at 223.
47 Lois Snyder (ed.), *Complementary and Alternative Medicine: Ethics, the Patient and the Physician*, Humana Press, Philadelphia, 2007, Wayne Vaught Chapter 3 pp. 45–75, 'Complementary and Alternative Medicine: The Physician's Ethical Obligations' at 48.
48 Ibid. at 51.
49 M. J. Johnstone, *Bioethics—A Nursing Perspective* (5th ed., 2009) Churchill Livingstone, Sydney, 2009, 67.
50 Beauchamp & Childress, *Principles of Biomedical Ethics*, 15.
51 Ibid., p. 68.
52 Weir, *Alternative Medicine: A New Regulatory Model*, Bond University Press, Gold Coast, 2005, 263.
53 Johnstone, Bioethics—A Nursing Perspective, 43–44.
54 K. Danner Clouser, David J Hufford & Bonnie Blair O'Connor, 'Informed Consent and Alternative Medicine' (1996) 2 *Alternative Therapies* 76–78; Stone & Matthews, above n. 3, 238–239.
55 M.H. Cohen, 'Legal and Ethical Issues in Complementary Medicine: A United States Perspective' (2004) 181 *Medical Journal of Australia* 168, where he discusses this dilemma from the perspective of a medical practitioner; and M.H. Cohen, 'Negotiating Integrative Medicine: A Framework for Provider–Patient Conversations' (2004) July *Negotiation Journal* 409, where he discusses principles of negotiation that may assist this process.
56 Lynoe, 'Ethical Professional Aspects', at 218.
57 House of Lords Science and Technology Committee, Sixth Report Session 1999–2000, para. 4.8.
58 J. Crellin & F. Ania, *Professionalism and Ethics in Complementary and Alternative Medicine*, Haworth Press, Binghampton, NY, 2001, p. 27.
59 Lynoe, 'Ethical Professional Aspects', at 218.
60 Crellin & Ania, *Professionalism and Ethics*, p. 27.
61 Beauchamp & Childress, *Principles of Biomedical Ethics*, p. 363.
62 Richards & Louise, *Medical Law and Ethics*, pp. 18–19.
63 Johnstone, *Bioethics—A Nursing Perspective*, p. 37.
64 Stone & Matthews, *Complementary Medicine and the Law*, p. 233.
65 https://www.ahpra.gov.au/Publications/Code-of-conduct.aspx (accessed 13 December 2021).
66 Johnstone, *Bioethics—A Nursing Perspective*, p. 21.
67 Coady & Bloch, *Codes of Ethics and the Professions*, p. 27.
68 Ibid., p. 83.
69 https://humanrights.gov.au/our-work/employers/quick-guide-australian-discrimination-laws (Accessed 20 August 2021).
70 Stone & Matthews, *Complementary Medicine and the Law*, p. 251.
71 www.osteopathyboard.gov.au/Codes-Guidelines.aspx; Refer also to Professional Boundaries Code of Conduct, https://www.chinesemedicineboard.gov.au/Codes-Guidelines/Code-of-conduct.aspx; para 8.2 (accessed 10 September 2021).
72 A. Dix et al., *Law for the Medical Profession*, Butterworths, Sydney, 1996, p. 403. 64.
73 Ibid., p. 67.
74 L. Campbell et al., *Risk Management in Chiropractic: Developing Risk Management Strategies*, Health Services Publication, Fincastle, VA, 1990, pp. 36–7.
75 *Tarasoff v Regents of the University of California* (1976) 17 Cal 3d 358. 68.
76 (1990) 1 All ER 835. Refer also to a Canadian case *Smith v Jones* [1999] 1 S.C.R. 455.
77 https://www.oaic.gov.au/privacy/privacy-in-your-state/ (accessed 2 September 2021).
78 https://www.oaic.gov.au/__data/assets/pdf_file/0011/2090/guide-to-health-privacy.pdf (accessed 2 September 2021).
79 https://www.oaic.gov.au/data/assets/pdf_filc/0011/2090/guide-to-health-privacy.pdf at Chapter 1 p. 1.
80 https://www.oaic.gov.au/privacy/guidance-and-advice/privacy-management-plan-template-for-organisations/ Chapter 1 p. 2.
81 https://www.oaic.gov.au/privacy/guidance-and-advice/privacy-management-plan-template-for-organisations/ Chapter 1 p. 2.

82   https://www.oaic.gov.au/privacy/guidance-and-advice/privacy-management-plan-template-for-organisations/ Chapter 1 p. 2.

83   https://www.oaic.gov.au/privacy/guidance-and-advice/privacy-management-plan-template-for-organisations/ Chapter 1 p. 5.

84   https://www.oaic.gov.au/privacy/guidance-and-advice/privacy-management-plan-template-for-organisations/ Chapter 2 p. 2.

85   https://www.oaic.gov.au/privacy/guidance-and-advice/privacy-management-plan-template-for-organisations/ Chapter 2 p. 2.

86   https://www.oaic.gov.au/privacy/guidance-and-advice/privacy-management-plan-template-for-organisations/ Chapter 2 p. 3.

87   https://www.oaic.gov.au/privacy/guidance-and-advice/privacy-management-plan-template-for-organisations/ Chapter 2 pp. 3, 4.

88   https://www.oaic.gov.au/privacy/guidance-and-advice/privacy-management-plan-template-for-organisations/ Chapter 2 p. 7.

89   https://www.oaic.gov.au/privacy/guidance-and-advice/privacy-management-plan-template-for-organisations/ Chapter 3 p. 2.

90   https://www.oaic.gov.au/privacy/guidance-and-advice/privacy-management-plan-template-for-organisations/ Chapter 3 p. 2.

91   https://www.oaic.gov.au/privacy/guidance-and-advice/privacy-management-plan-template-for-organisations/ Chapter 3 p. 3.

92   https://www.oaic.gov.au/privacy/guidance-and-advice/privacy-management-plan-template-for-organisations/

93   https://www.oaic.gov.au/privacy/guidance-and-advice/privacy-management-plan-template-for-organisations/ Chapter 3 p. 5.

94   https://www.oaic.gov.au/privacy/guidance-and-advice/privacy-management-plan-template-for-organisations/ Chapter 4 p. 1.

95   https://www.oaic.gov.au/privacy/guidance-and-advice/privacy-management-plan-template-for-organisations/ Chapter 4 p. 3.

96   https://www.oaic.gov.au/privacy/guidance-and-advice/privacy-management-plan-template-for-organisations/ Chapter 4 p. 5.

97   https://www.oaic.gov.au/privacy/guidance-and-advice/privacy-management-plan-template-for-organisations/ Chapter 4 p. 8.

98   https://www.oaic.gov.au/privacy/guidance-and-advice/privacy-management-plan-template-for-organisations/ Chapter 5 p. 2.

99   https://www.oaic.gov.au/privacy/guidance-and-advice/privacy-management-plan-template-for-organisations/ Chapter 6 p. 1.

100 https://www.oaic.gov.au/privacy/guidance-and-advice/privacy-management-plan-template-for-organisations/ Chapter 6 p. 2.

101 https://www.oaic.gov.au/privacy/guidance-and-advice/privacy-management-plan-template-for-organisations/ Chapter 7 p. 1.

102 https://www.oaic.gov.au/privacy/guidance-and-advice/privacy-management-plan-template-for-organisations/ Chapter 8 p. 1.

103 https://www.oaic.gov.au/privacy/guidance-and-advice/privacy-management-plan-template-for-organisations/ Chapter 9 p. 1.

104 https://www.oaic.gov.au/privacy/guidance-and-advice/privacy-management-plan-template-for-organisations/ Chapter 9 pp. 1–2.

105 Stone & Matthews, *Complementary Medicine and the Law*, p. 263.

106 Under section15 of the *Oranga Tamariki Act 1989 Children, Young People's Well-being Act 1981*.

107 J. McIlwraith & W. Madden, *Health Care and the Law*, 6th ed., Thomson Reuters, Sydney, 2014, p. 579.

108 J. Edgington (ed.), *Law for the Nursing Profession*, 3rd ed., CCH, Sydney, 1995, p. 109.

109 J.D. Harrison, *Chiropractic Practice Liability: A Practical Guide to Successful Risk Management*, International Chiropractors' Association, Arlington, VA, 1990, p. 64.

110 [2004] SADC 190 (22 December 2004).

111 National Law, s 178.

112 *Romeo v Asher* (1991) 29 FCR 343.

113 *Kioa v West* (1985) 159 CLR 550 at 585, 612.
114 www.ahpra.gov.au/Notifications/mandatorynotifications/Mandatory-notifications.aspx (accessed 15 August 2021).
115 J. Forbes, *Justice in Tribunals*, 4th ed., Federation Press, Sydney, 2014, p. 2.
116 Ibid., p. 3. 82.
117 Ibid., p. 76. 83.
118 Ibid., p. 80. 84.
119 Ibid., p. 75.
120 Ibid., p. 98.
121 Ibid., pp. 129–50.
122 Ibid., pp. 170–1.
123 Ibid., p. 171.
124 Ibid., pp. 151–65.
125 Ibid., p. 254.
126 Ibid., p. 234.
127 Ibid., p. 251.

4 Restricted acts and protected titles

A health professional uses all available techniques to resolve the health concerns of a client. This legitimate aim does not permit a practitioner to perform acts called 'restricted acts'[1] that must only be performed by specified registered health professionals. Penalties may also apply to unregistered practitioners who are representing that they are registered or using protected titles that must only be used by registered professionals.

A breach of the National Law might occur where:

- a practitioner performs a restricted act that they are not entitled to perform, such as manipulation of the cervical spine, or
- a practitioner breaches the 'holding out' provisions of professional registration statutes.

Ignorance of these parameters can result in:

- action by one of the national registration boards, such as the Chiropractic Board of Australia which have considerable penalties including criminal penalties.
- the voiding of professional indemnity insurance, and
- professional misconduct proceedings.

Chiropractors, osteopaths and Chinese medicine practitioners, acupuncturists and Chinese herbal medicine dispensers are the only registered complementary medicine practitioners in Australia. These practitioners need to understand their relationship with other registered professions.

BOX 4.1

Action plan

- Do not use titles, marketing or advertising that will incorrectly suggest that you are a medical doctor or any other registered health professional.
- Do not perform restricted acts limited to specified registered health professionals.
- Refer clients to a medical practitioner or other health professional when a health issue relates to a matter outside your scope of practice.

DOI: 10.4324/9781003195931-4

National health practitioner legislation

The National Registration and Accreditation Scheme for Health Professions commenced on 1 July 2010, based upon an agreement between the states and territories to provide for a single national registration and accreditation scheme for health professions. The health professions included in the national scheme are currently chiropractic, dental, medical, nursing and midwifery, optometry, osteopathy, pharmacy, physiotherapy, podiatry and psychology, Aboriginal and Torres Strait Islander health practice, Chinese medicine, medical radiation, paramedicine and occupational therapy.

Queensland hosted the substantive legislation to give effect to the national scheme, with other jurisdictions enacting identical legislation other than essential local provisions. The *Health Practitioner Regulation National Law Act 2009* (Qld) was enacted on 3 November 2009 by the Queensland Parliament, and all other jurisdictions have enacted the required legislation that generally mirrors that legislation.[2] As each state has enacted almost identical legislation with the same section numbering for most provisions to reflect the national scheme, in this chapter reference to sections of the legislation will be described as sections of the 'National Law'.

This reform means that the system of registration and accreditation of health professions is similar though not identical in each jurisdiction, allowing the application of national standards and accreditation requirements. In New South Wales there are substantial changes to the National Law in relation to health performance and conduct (refer to *Health Practitioner Regulation National Law Act 2009* (NSW) (refer to Schedule 1) and the creation in that state of professional councils such as the Osteopathy Council of New South Wales to work with the national board. In addition, Queensland has a co-regulatory jurisdiction, co-regulatory authority and the adjudication body (Health Ombudsman) for dealing with health, performance and conduct process.[3] The national scheme has resulted in most individual state health profession registration boards being replaced by a single national board for each registered health profession. For example, the Chiropractic Board of Australia will serve all chiropractors throughout all jurisdictions in Australia to replace each state registration board subject to the New South Wales and Queensland legislative amendments.

Role of national boards

Each national board consists of a chair who is a member of the relevant profession with at least 50 per cent of the remaining members from the relevant profession and no more than two thirds of the board being members of the profession. The board has a role that includes development of competency and accreditation standards; approval of accredited courses; decisions on registration applications; and overseeing receipt and investigation of complaints against registered practitioners, including referral of serious matters for hearing by relevant external tribunals or disciplinary processes for less serious matters.

'Holding out' as a health practitioner

Consumers are entitled to understand the nature of the services that a practitioner will provide. Division 10 of the National Law provides that it is an offence for a person to use a 'protected title' unless he or she is the specific registered health professional who is entitled to use that protected title. Advertising, marketing, signage and literature should avoid any suggestion that a practitioner is entitled to use a protected title unless they are entitled to use that title, or use any word, symbol or device that might suggest that they are a registered health practitioner.

A person must not knowingly or recklessly take or use a title or use a protected title for a health profession that could reasonably be expected to induce a belief that the person or another person is registered under the National Law for a health profession unless they are registered for that profession. This prohibition applies whether the title is used with other words and whether in English or another language. The protected titles relevant to the registered health professions are shown in Table 4.1.

Table 4.1 Protected titles for registered health professions

Profession	*Title*
Aboriginal and Torres Strait Islander health practice	Aboriginal and Torres Strait Islander health practitioner, Aboriginal health practitioner, Torres Strait Islander health practitioner
Chinese medicine	Chinese medicine practitioner, Chinese herbal dispenser, Chinese herbal medicine practitioner, Oriental medicine practitioner, acupuncturist
Chiropractic	Chiropractor
Dental	Dentist, dental therapist, dental hygienist, dental prosthetist, oral health therapist
Medical	Medical practitioner
Medical radiation practice	Medical radiation practitioner, diagnostic radiographer, medical imaging technologist, radiographer, nuclear medicine scientist, nuclear medicine technologist, radiation therapist
Nursing and midwifery	Nurse, registered nurse, nurse practitioner, enrolled nurse, midwife, midwife practitioner
Occupational therapy	Occupational therapist
Optometry	Optometrist, optician
Osteopathy	Osteopath
Paramedicine	Paramedic
Pharmacy	Pharmacist, pharmaceutical chemist
Physiotherapy	Physiotherapist, physical therapist
Podiatry	Podiatrist, chiropodist
Psychology	Psychologist

Provision is made for some registered health practitioners not registered for Chinese Medicine to be endorsed to use the title 'acupuncturist' pursuant to section 97 of the National Law if they are qualified. If so endorsed, that person does not breach the above provisions in relation to the use of that title. Currently about 600 medical doctors are so endorsed in regard to using the title of acupuncturist.

The National Law also restricts the use of the title 'dental specialist', 'medical specialist' or a specialist title for a recognised speciality unless the person is registered as a specialist.[4] Also restricted is the use of the titles such as 'registered health practitioner' and 'specialist health practitioner', or the use of a title, name, initial, symbol, word or description that could reasonably be understood to indicate that the person is a health practitioner or a specialist health practitioner; or the person is authorised or qualified to practise in a health profession or as a specialist health practitioner; or claim to be registered under this law or hold himself or herself out as being registered under the National Law.[5] This could include the use of terms such as 'surgeon' or 'doctor' where it might be seen as a representation that the person or another person is a registered health professional. The most obvious offences relate to holding out or using titles or other words indicating a person is a medical practitioner, a chiropractor or an osteopath.[6]

These provisions are complex, and it is not intended to deal with every potential breach of these holding-out provisions in this chapter. What is clear from these provisions is that practitioners must ensure that they market themselves accurately and do not represent that they have statutory endorsement they do not possess. Additionally, practitioners should not use words or symbols that might reasonably be interpreted to mean that they are a registered health practitioner or a specific type of registered health practitioner when they do not enjoy that status. This might occur if a person who is not a registered physiotherapist uses the term 'physio' to describe their practice.

In regard to the issue of holding out as a registered health practitioner in breach of the National Law, a decision in *Penev v County Court* (Vic) provides some clarification. This involved an action by the Chinese Medicine Registration Board of Victoria under the *Health Professions Registration Act 2005* (HPRA) before the passing of the National Law but the statute was similar.[7] Ms Pevel brought a Supreme Court appeal against a County Court decision that Ms Pevel, a naturopath, was in breach of the HPRA for applying 'laser acupuncture' that demonstrated a 'holding out' as a registered health practitioner. Although using the protected title 'acupuncturist' would breach the HPRA (and the National law provisions) it was accepted by Emerton J of the Victorian Supreme Court that using the word 'acupuncture' or the actual practice of acupuncture was not a breach by itself. What might be a breach was a breach of the section 80 of HPRA.

Section 80 HPRA

Claims by persons as to registration

(1) A person who is not a registered health practitioner must not intentionally or recklessly—

   (b) take or use a title, name, initial, symbol, word or description that, having regard to the circumstances in which it is taken or used, indicates or could be reasonably understood to indicate—

      (i) the person is a health practitioner in a regulated health profession; or

   (c) claim to be registered under this Act or hold himself or herself out as being registered under this Act;

The County Court decision suggested that Ms Penev used words which could reasonably be understood to indicate that she was an acupuncturist when she was not registered with the Board, because her website suggested she was qualified to assist with a range of health issues with a speciality in laser acupuncture. Ms Penev was also said to have held herself out as being registered as an acupuncturist when she was not registered with the Board, because she conducted an acupuncture consultation and represented that she could provide laser acupuncture services. It was alleged that by advertising and/or providing 'laser acupuncture', she held herself out to be a registered practitioner under the HPRA.[8]

Emerton J of the Victorian Supreme Court concluded that in regard to the HPRA the 'regulatory regime was based, not on prohibitions or restrictions on the actual performance of acupuncture, but on prohibitions or restrictions on the practitioner claiming or holding out that he or she was registered or endorsed by a responsible Board to perform acupuncture. The regulatory regime was, as the defendant submits, largely based on title protection.'[9]

The appeal by Ms Penev to the Supreme Court against the County Court conviction was successful on the basis that the County Court did not 'analyse the factual evidence to determine whether the conduct of Penev could reasonably be understood to induce a belief that the person was registered under the HPRA'.[10] This meant the County Court did not fully deal with the issue of whether a non-registered health practitioner who does not use the restricted title but applies the techniques of the modality such as using Chinese herbs is in breach of the HPRA.

Although the practitioner was successful in this authority, the nature of the discussion in the *Pevel* case does require caution for practitioners. If a statement is made by a health practitioner such as a naturopath to a client 'I am going to give you a Chinese Medicine herb used by TCM practitioners' this may reasonably suggest the practitioner is holding out as a Chinese medicine practitioner and might suggest the circumstances are in breach of the National Law.[11] If a herb is identified as TCM herbs and is applied for a client along with other non-TCM remedies it may indicate the herb is part of naturopathic practice involving various forms of therapy and not holding out as a TCM practitioner.[12]

It is suggested 'A practitioner should avoid indicating they are practising TCM involving the prescription of a TCM substance. It may be advisable to limit prescription to pre-prepared herbs rather than using a TCM dispenser or with raw herbs as this may more easily tend to suggest the practitioner is acting as a TCM registered practitioner.'[13]

In addition 'Advertising, stationery, letterhead, website entries and discussions with clients should not include words or other indications that might reasonably suggest that the practitioner is a registered health practitioner or authorised or qualified to practise as a registered health practitioner.'[14]

One title sometimes used in the context of Chinese medicine and acupuncture treatment by unregistered health practitioners or by physiotherapists as an adjunct to their standard practices is 'dry needling'. This term is not protected by the National Law. The question of whether this therapy is in fact acupuncture by another name is a complex issue but currently the use of that term does not by itself result in a breach of the National Law, though a consumer should question the level of training undertaken by the practitioners of this modality as against registered Chinese medicine practitioners.[15]

BOX 4.2

Practice tip

A cautious practitioner wishing to avoid possible scrutiny under the provisions discussed above would consider taking the following precautions:

- In your marketing, stationery and phone book entries, limit your entries to name, phone number, email and/or web address, postal address, modality or modalities and professional associations. For example:

  - John James, Naturopath,
  - Bach Flower Remedies, Aromatherapy
  - Address: 17 Webb Road Edenville
  - Telephone no: 5467850
  - Email address: jamesnaturopath@dinki.com.au
  - Member Gold Coast Association of Naturopaths

- If you mention particular diseases, do not hold out or represent that you can cure those diseases
- In advertisements, never use words, terms or devices (such as a stethoscope, hypodermic needle or 'physio') that might be construed as indicating that you are a registered health practitioner; don't use the terms 'surgeon', 'specialist', 'doctor' or 'physician' (even if used with 'natural medicine' or 'Chinese'). Chiropractors and osteopaths may be able to use the term 'doctor' if the qualifier 'chiropractic', 'chiropractor', 'osteopathy' or 'osteopath' is attached (see discussion at page 211). Refer also to AHPRA, Guidelines for Advertising Regulated Health Service, December 2020.

It should be remembered that any holding out is based on what someone other than yourself might perceive you to be. If you have a doctorate, such as a Doctor of Philosophy degree, the nature of the doctorate should be explained to avoid confusion.

Practice provisions: restricted acts

The National Law creates offences for unregistered persons undertaking specified activities, and describes three restricted acts that must only be performed by medical practitioners or specified registered health professions. These acts are:

- restricted dental acts[16]
- prescribing optical appliances,[17] and
- performing manipulation of the cervical spine.[18]

In this book, the focus will be on the restricted act being performing manipulation of the cervical spine. Section 123 provides as follows:

1 A person must not perform manipulation of the cervical spine unless the person:

   a is registered in an appropriate health profession; or
   b is a student who performs manipulation of the cervical spine in the course of activities undertaken as part of—

      i an approved program of study in an appropriate health profession; or
      ii clinical training in an appropriate health profession; or

2 is a person, or a member of a class of persons, prescribed under a regulation as being authorised to perform manipulation of the cervical spine.

Maximum penalty—$60,000 or 3 years of imprisonment or both.

In this section, appropriate health profession means any of the following health professions—

a   chiropractic
b   osteopathy
c   medical
d   physiotherapy.

'Manipulation of the cervical spine' means moving the joints of the cervical spine beyond a person's usual physiological range of motion using a high-velocity, low-amplitude thrust.

It is only the manipulation of the cervical spine that is restricted. The cervical spine is normally defined to include the neck region of the spine containing the first seven vertebrae.[19]

This provision limits the performance of manipulation of the cervical spine to chiropractors, osteopaths, medical practitioners and physiotherapists. Manipulation of the cervical spine by persons other than these appropriate health professions would involve a breach of these provisions. Note that the maximum penalty for such an offence is $60,000 or 3 years of imprisonment or both. This is particularly relevant for practitioners of therapeutic massage, touch for health therapists, shiatsu and other similar modalities that may deal with related procedures.

What is manipulation?

In a South Australian District Court case, *Edwards v Butler*,[20] the issue of what constitutes a 'manipulation' was discussed. The judge did not clearly define the term in the judgement but he appears to have accepted the definition of the term provided by two chiropractor expert witnesses. One expert suggested that a 'manipulation' was 'an application of force in a particular direction resulting in joint cavitation' with the 'accompanying cracking sound which he said is the signature that a manipulation has taken place'.[21] The other expert suggested 'that a joint manipulation with a "crack" (cavitation) is well defined in the literature as being where the range of motion of a joint is taken into the paraphysiological zone, usually with a high velocity, low amplitude thrust'.[22] This expert chiropractor also suggested that occasionally during soft tissue management a joint may crack without any intention on the part of the practitioner.[23] There is nothing in the judgement to suggest that this unintentional 'crack' should be deemed a manipulation.

High-velocity manipulation

The restricted act in section 123 of the National Law relates to moving the joints of the cervical spine beyond a person's usual physiological range of motion using a high-velocity, low-amplitude thrust. This would suggest that low-velocity manipulation would not breach this provision. How one differentiates between low- and high-velocity manipulation in a practical situation is a moot point. The limited nature of this restricted act described in section 123 of the National Law appears to be a less problematic form of regulation for complementary medicine practitioners than applied under prior legislation. A breach of section 123 would appear to require proof that:

- the joints of the cervical spine were moved, and
- this movement is beyond a person's usual physiological range of motion, and
- the movement was caused by a high-velocity, low-amplitude thrust, and
- the above acts were completed by a person who is not a registered chiropractor, osteopath, medical practitioner or physiotherapist.

Intended manipulation

A practitioner who applies a technique with the intention of manipulating the cervical spine may breach this provision if the manipulation is high velocity with a low-amplitude thrust. If the practitioner is not an authorised practitioner, this activity will likely be deemed an offence.

Unintended manipulation

A practitioner of therapeutic massage or other similar modality may indirectly or unintentionally cause a manipulation or adjustment of the cervical spine. The terminology used in section 123 of the National Law may suggest that the prohibition relates to purposeful or intended manipulation or adjustment of the cervical spine. Although it is difficult to determine how this provision will be interpreted, it is suggested that it is unlikely section 123 of the National Law would penalise unintended and indirect manipulation of the cervical spine that sometimes arises during massage and manual therapy not directed to the cervical spine or performed on the cervical spine area without any intention to cause a manipulation. Great care should be taken when providing therapy to the cervical spine to avoid arguments that a manipulation of that area is contemplated or sought.

   An issue may arise if a manipulation occurs for part of the spine near to the cervical spine, which causes an associated adjustment to the cervical spine. One would advise a practitioner to only manipulate the spine if they have proper training in that procedure and it would be advisable to ensure that the procedures will not indirectly cause a manipulation of the cervical spine in breach of this provision.

New Zealand provisions

In New Zealand, the *Health Practitioners Competence Assurance Act 2003* (HPCAA) regulates the provision of health services by registered health practitioners.[24] This is omnibus legislation that covers all registered health professions, including chiropractors, osteopaths, dentists, dieticians, medical doctors, medical radiation technologists, midwives, nurses, occupational therapists, optometrists, pharmacists, paramedics, podiatry, psychology, psychotherapy and physiotherapists.

   The HPCAA creates 'holding out' offences for persons not entitled to use a specific title, the description of a scope of practice for registered health professions and specific restricted activities limited to registered health practitioners who have that practice within their scope of practice.

Holding out

Section 7 of the HPCAA provides that a person may only use names, words, titles, initials, abbreviations or descriptions stating or implying that the person is a health practitioner of a particular kind if that person is registered and is qualified to be registered as a health practitioner of that kind. This would require a medical doctor, chiropractor or osteopath to be duly registered to allow them to use a title such as 'MD', 'chiropractor' or 'osteopath' that might suggest they are registered for that profession. This provision does not specify which titles or words are restricted to specific registered health professions.

Scope of practice: general comments

Section 8 of the HPCAA states that no health practitioner may perform a health service that forms part of a scope of practice of the profession unless that practitioner is permitted to perform that service by his or her scope of practice and performs that service in accordance with any conditions stated in that scope of practice. This provision is directed primarily to ensure a health practitioner only performs an act within the described scope of practice for the health profession if they are permitted to do that act under the scope of practice and in accordance with any stated conditions.

The *Guidelines for the Operation of Restricted Activities under the Health Practitioners Competence Assurance Act 2003* provide some useful information. Section 11 of the HPCAA requires each registered health profession to specify a scope of practice by Gazette. This has occurred under the *New Zealand Gazette* ('the Gazette') no. 120, 30 June 2005, involving scope of practice for all the registered health professions including chiropractic and osteopathy.

Restricted activities

Section 9 of the HPCAA states that the Governor-General may by Order in Council declare an activity that constitutes or forms part of a health service to be a restricted activity. Under section 9(4) of the HPCAA, no person may perform or state or imply that he or she is willing to perform an activity that by an Order in Council made under this section is declared to be a restricted activity unless the person is a health practitioner who is permitted by his or her scope of practice to perform that activity. The Health Practitioners Competence Assurance (Restricted Activities) Order 2005 Schedule contains five restricted activities:

1 Surgical or operative procedures below the gingival margin or the surface of the skin, mucous membranes, or teeth.
2 Clinical procedures involved in the insertion and maintenance of fixed and removable orthodontic or oral and maxillofacial prosthetic appliances.
3 Prescribing of enteral or parenteral nutrition where the feed is administered through a tube into the gut or central venous catheter.
4 Prescribing of an ophthalmic appliance, optical appliance, or ophthalmic medical device intended for remedial or cosmetic purposes or for the correction of a defect of sight.
5 Applying high-velocity, low-amplitude manipulative techniques to cervical spinal joints.

Of most relevance to complementary medicine practitioners is the provision limiting high-velocity, low-amplitude manipulative techniques to cervical spinal joints. This description reflects generally the Australian restricted act in relation to manipulation of the cervical spine. The discussion above in relation to how this technique should be defined is relevant.

One query might arise in relation to restricted activity no. 1 in relation to acupuncture, which will involve insertion of acupuncture needles below the surface of the skin. The reference to 'surgical or operative procedures' would seem to suggest that acupuncture does not breach this provision. The *Guidelines for the Operation of Restricted Activities under the Health Practitioners Competence Assurance Act 2003* state with regard to restricted activity no. 1[25]:

> This is intended to broadly capture activities that involve cutting the flesh or doing something that causes bleeding. Particular reference is made to teeth and to the gingival margin (the 'gum'). [NB In many cases, evidence of bleeding will give rise to a presumption of an offence. The Ministry would take note of the occurrence of blood or bleeding as a result of actions taken by non-registered individuals when considering if a breach of this restricted activity has occurred. If it appears that a breach has occurred, the occurrence of blood/bleeding will be taken as evidence of a breach of this restricted activity].

Scope of practice provisions

The scope of practice of the registered health professions under the Gazette deal generally with the restricted activities specified above. In relation to chiropractic, there is reference in the scope of practice for that profession to 'utilise chiropractic adjustment(s) and/or manipulation(s)', which would cover restricted activity no. 5 above.

The scope of practice for osteopathy makes a more general reference to 'osteopathic manipulative techniques [that] are taught in the core curricula of accredited courses in osteopathy'. Note that the scope of practice for osteopathy is currently under review. Refer to the Osteopathic Scope of Practice Reform.[26] There is also a scope of practice for osteopaths using Western medical acupuncture and related needling techniques.

The *Guidelines for the Operation of Restricted Activities under the Health Practitioners Competence Assurance Act 2003* state[27]:

> The restricted activities do not, in themselves, limit what activities a registered health practitioner may carry out. Under the Act the activity of practitioners is determined by the scopes of practice within which they work. A registered health practitioner may do anything in his or her scope of practice—including an activity that is otherwise restricted if that scope of practice covers or clearly includes that activity. It is not necessary for a scope of practice to specifically refer to a restricted activity; only that the scope clearly countenances it. A health practitioner who acts outside his or her scope of practice will be subject to proceedings initiated by his or her registration authority.

The Guidelines also state[28]:

> It was recognised that the wording should not inadvertently capture existing lawful and safe activities. For example, the following activities are not considered by the Ministry to be captured by the listed restricted activities:
>
> * acupuncture
> * taking blood samples
> * the manufacture of a customised anti-snoring device
> * taking of dental impressions (for example, for the production of mouth guards)
> * minor tasks and simple procedures undertaken by caregivers, such as lancing of boils or pulling out loose teeth, and
> * making and fitting of ocular prosthetics.

The structure of this legislation suggests that registered health practitioners need to ensure that their practice complies with the statutory scope of practice as it is currently determined, noting that they need to establish that this scope of practice covers any restricted acts. One would imagine that standard professional practice will in most cases comply with these requirements.

With regard to unregistered complementary medicine practitioners—such as acupuncturists, massage therapists and homoeopaths—they need to ensure that they do not perform restricted acts in their practice and are best served by keeping within the standard scope of practice for their profession.

Codes of conduct for unregistered health practitioners

Concern has been expressed in Australia with regard to the activities of some unregistered health professionals, including formerly registered health professionals who now practise in related fields after being suspended or deregistered. The discipline and enforcement provisions available under registration statutes are not available to stop some unfair, unethical, criminal and dangerous practices by a small proportion of unregistered health practitioners. This gap in the legislation and a number of concerning cases of unethical and dangerous acts by unregistered health practitioners led to New South Wales, Victoria, Queensland and South Australia enacting a Code of Conduct for Unregistered Health Practitioners to regulate the activities of those health workers, giving powers to grant prohibition orders against their activities.[29]

These Codes of Conduct are a form of 'negative licensing', which means there are limited controls on entry into the industry but they provide a power to prohibit a person from practising in some areas, or to prohibit practice entirely based upon a breach of the relevant Code.

Such concerns and the success of the New South Wales Code of Conduct prompted a review of this issue by the Australian Health Ministers' Advisory Council (AHMAC). This culminated in a decision by the COAG Health Council in April 2015 to establish a National Code of Conduct for Health Care Workers, similar but not the same as the New South Wales example, to be enacted in all jurisdictions in Australia. Refer to the COAG final report, *A National Code of Conduct for Healthcare Workers*, 17 April 2015 (COAG Final Report) in relation to the details of this proposed National Code of Conduct.[30]

The expectation that there would be a national code of conduct in place has not yet been realised. Currently New South Wales, Victoria, Queensland and South Australia have enacted a Code of Conduct. Tasmania has passed legislation including a Code of Conduct but it has not yet been enacted.[31] Western Australia, Australian Capital Territory and Northern Territory have not yet completed a Code of Conduct reflecting the National Code.

New South Wales Code

Section 100 of the *Public Health Act 2010* (NSW) provides that regulations may prescribe codes of conduct for the provision of health services by unregistered health practitioners (including deregistered health practitioners) and registered health practitioners who provide health services that are unrelated to their registration.

Schedule 3 of the *Public Health (General) Regulation 2012* (NSW) contains the Code of Conduct, which relates to the provision of health services, including services provided by chiropractors, osteopaths, masseurs, naturopaths, acupuncturists and those in other alternative healthcare fields. Accordingly, these regulations deal with most, if not all, complementary medicine practitioners.

The New South Wales Code of Conduct contains sixteen conduct requirements of which practitioners should be aware in their practice. Most are behaviours that normally would be followed by any competent and ethical practitioner; however, it does raise issues that may impact on the approach taken in some significant areas. The Code of Conduct https://www.health.nsw.gov.au/phact/Pages/code-of-conduct.aspx includes the following provisions relevant to complementary medicine practice:

3 Health practitioners to provide services in safe and ethical manner

1 A health practitioner must provide health services in a safe and ethical manner.
2 Without limiting subclause (1), health practitioners must comply with the following principles:

   a a health practitioner must maintain the necessary competence in his or her field of practice,
   b a health practitioner must not provide health care of a type that is outside his or her experience or training,
   c a health practitioner must not provide services that he or she is not qualified to provide,
   d a health practitioner must not use his or her possession of particular qualifications to mislead or deceive his or her clients as to his or her competence in his or her field of practice or ability to provide treatment,
   e a health practitioner must prescribe only treatments or appliances that serve the needs of the client,
   f a health practitioner must recognise the limitations of the treatment he or she can provide and refer clients to other competent health practitioners in appropriate circumstances,
   g a health practitioner must recommend to his or her clients that additional opinions and services be sought, where appropriate,

    h   a health practitioner must assist his or her clients to find other appropriate health care professionals, if required and practicable,

    i   a health practitioner must encourage his or her clients to inform their treating medical practitioner (if any) of the treatments they are receiving,

    j   a health practitioner must have a sound understanding of any adverse interactions between the therapies and treatments he or she provides or prescribes and any other medications or treatments, whether prescribed or not, that the health practitioner is aware the client is taking or receiving,

    k   a health practitioner must ensure that appropriate first aid is available to deal with any misadventure during a client consultation,

    l   a health practitioner must obtain appropriate emergency assistance (for example, from the Ambulance Service) in the event of any serious misadventure during a client consultation.

4 Health practitioners diagnosed with infectious medical condition

1 A health practitioner who has been diagnosed with a medical condition that can be passed on to clients must ensure that he or she practises in a manner that does not put clients at risk.

2 Without limiting subclause (1), a health practitioner who has been diagnosed with a medical condition that can be passed on to clients should take and follow advice from an appropriate medical practitioner on the steps to be taken to modify his or her practice to avoid the possibility of transmitting that condition to clients.

5 Health practitioners not to make claims to cure certain serious illnesses

1 A health practitioner must not hold himself or herself out as qualified, able or willing to cure cancer and other terminal illnesses.

2 A health practitioner may make a claim as to his or her ability or willingness to treat or alleviate the symptoms of those illnesses if that claim can be substantiated.

6 Health practitioners to adopt standard precautions for infection control

1 A health practitioner must adopt standard precautions for the control of infection in his or her practice.

2 Without limiting subclause (1), a health practitioner who carries out a skin penetration procedure must comply with the relevant regulations of this Regulation in relation to the carrying out of the procedure.[32]

7 Appropriate conduct in relation to treatment advice

1 A health practitioner must not attempt to dissuade clients from seeking or continuing with treatment by a registered medical practitioner.

2 A health practitioner must accept the right of his or her clients to make informed choices in relation to their health care.

3 A health practitioner should communicate and co-operate with colleagues and other health care practitioners and agencies in the best interests of their clients.

4 A health practitioner who has serious concerns about the treatment provided to any of his or her clients by another health practitioner must refer the matter to the Health Care Complaints Commission.

8 Health practitioners not to practise under influence of alcohol or drugs

1 A health practitioner must not practise under the influence of alcohol or unlawful drugs.
2 A health practitioner who is taking prescribed medication must obtain advice from the prescribing health practitioner on the impact of the medication on his or her ability to practise and must refrain from treating clients in circumstances where his or her ability is or may be impaired.

9 Health practitioners not to practise with certain physical or mental conditions

A health practitioner must not practise while suffering from a physical or mental impairment, disability, condition or disorder (including an addiction to alcohol or a drug, whether or not prescribed) that detrimentally affects, or is likely to detrimentally affect, his or her ability to practise or that places clients at risk of harm.

10 Health practitioners not to financially exploit clients

1 A health practitioner must not accept financial inducements or gifts for referring clients to other health practitioners or to the suppliers of medications or therapeutic goods or devices.
2 A health practitioner must not offer financial inducements or gifts in return for client referrals from other health practitioners.
3 A health practitioner must not provide services and treatments to clients unless they are designed to maintain or improve the clients' health or wellbeing.

11 Health practitioners required to have clinical basis for treatments

A health practitioner must not diagnose or treat an illness or condition without an adequate clinical basis.

12 Health practitioners not to misinform their clients

1 A health practitioner must not engage in any form of misinformation or misrepresentation in relation to the products or services he or she provides or as to his or her qualifications, training or professional affiliations.
2 A health practitioner must provide truthful information as to his or her qualifications, training or professional affiliations if asked by a client.
3 A health practitioner must not make claims, either directly or in advertising or promotional material, about the efficacy of treatment or services provided if those claims cannot be substantiated.

13 Health practitioners not to engage in sexual or improper personal relationship with client

1 A health practitioner must not engage in a sexual or other close personal relationship with a client.
2 Before engaging in a sexual or other close personal relationship with a former client, a health practitioner must ensure that a suitable period of time has elapsed since the conclusion of their therapeutic relationship.

Note the examples of sexual behaviour discussed at page 43 of the COAG Final Report, namely sexual, personal or erotic comments,

- comments about a person's private life, sexuality or the way they look
- sexually suggestive comments or jokes
- repeated requests to go out
- requests for sex
- sexually explicit emails, text messages or posts on social networking sites
- inappropriate touching, including with the implication that is has a therapeutic benefit
- not charging or billing for treatment, unrelated to financial hardship.

14 Health practitioners to comply with relevant privacy laws

A health practitioner must comply with the relevant legislation of the State or the Commonwealth relating to his or her clients' health information, including the Commonwealth *Privacy Act 1988* and the New South Wales *Health Records and Information Privacy Act* 2002.

15 Health practitioners to keep appropriate records

A health practitioner must maintain accurate, legible and contemporaneous clinical records for each client consultation.

16 Health practitioners to keep appropriate insurance

A health practitioner should ensure that appropriate indemnity insurance arrangements are in place in relation to his or her practice.

17 Certain health practitioners to display code and other information

1 A health practitioner must display a copy of each of the following documents at all premises where the health practitioner carries on his or her practice:

  a   this code of Conduct,
  b   a document that gives information about the way in which clients may make a complaint to the Health Care Complaints Commission, being a document in a form approved by the Secretary.

2 Copies of those documents must be displayed in a position and manner that makes them easily visible to clients entering the relevant premises.
3 This clause does not apply to any of the following premises:

  a   the premises of any body within the public health system (as defined in section 6 of the *Health Services Act 1997*),
  b   private hospitals or day procedure centres (as defined in the *Private Hospitals and Day Procedure Centres Act 1988*),
  c   premises of the Ambulance Service of NSW (as defined in the *Health Services Act 1997*),
  d   premises of approved providers (within the meaning of the *Aged Care Act 1997* of the Commonwealth).

18 Sale and supply of optical appliances

Likely not relevant to complementary medicine.

Powers to grant prohibitions orders

The four Codes of Conduct have in place provision for warnings and interim or continuing prohibition orders or a public statement in the case of a person which has breached the terms of the Code of Conduct. Pursuant to section 41A–41E of the New South Wales *Health Care Complaints Act 1993*, the Health Care Complaints Commission can make a prohibition order against a registered or an unregistered practitioner. This is possible where, after proper investigation, the Commission finds that the health care practitioner has breached a code of conduct for unregistered health practitioners or has been convicted of a relevant offence and it thinks the health practitioner poses a substantial risk to the health of members of the public. The prohibition order can prohibit specified health services for a period of time or prohibit all provision of health services by that practitioner.

Pursuant to section 94A of the *Health Care Complaints Act 1993*, the Commission, after investigation, may cause a public statement to be issued or provide warnings about a treatment or health service if it considers it poses a risk to public health or safety. Similar provisions are found in the South Australian *Health and Community Services Complaints Act 2004* s 56B–56D.

A number of prohibition orders and public statements have been issued in New South Wales in relation to health practitioners, the details of which can be found at https://www.hccc.nsw.gov.au/Decisions.

Victoria, Queensland and South Australia National Code of Conduct for Health Care Workers

Victoria, Queensland and South Australia have enacted a Code of Conduct for Health Care Workers which are virtually identical other than the inserted local statutes and the definition of the applicable health practitioner subject to the Code. For the Victorian Code the reference is to a 'general health service provider'[33] while Qld and South Australia apply the term 'health care worker'.[34] This discussion is of the Queensland Code of Conduct for Health Care Workers. https://www.health.qld.gov.au/_data/assets/pdf_file/0014/444101/national-code-conduct-health-workers.pdf

Definitions

In this code of conduct:

- health care worker means a natural person who provides a health service (whether or not the person is registered under the Health Practitioner Regulation National Law)
- health service has the same meaning as in Section 7 of the *Health Ombudsman Act 2013* (Qld).

Application of code of conduct

This code of conduct applies to the provision of health services by:

a   health care workers who are not required to be registered under the Health Practitioner Regulation National Law (including de-registered health practitioners), and
b   health care workers who are registered health practitioners under the Health Practitioner Regulation National Law and who provide health services that are unrelated to their registration.

1   Health care workers to provide services in a safe and ethical manner

1   A health care worker must provide health services in a safe and ethical manner.
2   Without limiting subclause 1, health care workers must comply with the following:

   a   A health care worker must maintain the necessary competence in his or her field of practice
   b   A health care worker must not provide health care of a type that is outside his or her experience or training, or provide services that he or she is not qualified to provide
   c   A health care worker must only prescribe or recommend treatments or appliances that serve the needs of clients
   d   A health care worker must recognise the limitations of the treatment he or she can provide and refer clients to other competent health service providers in appropriate circumstances
   e   A health care worker must recommend to clients that additional opinions and services be sought, where appropriate
   f   A health care worker must assist a client to find other appropriate health care services, if required and practicable
   g   A health care worker must encourage clients to inform their treating medical practitioner (if any) of the treatments or care being provided
   h   A health care worker must have a sound understanding of any possible adverse interactions between the therapies and treatments being provided or prescribed and any other medications or treatments, whether prescribed or not, that he or she is, or should be, aware that a client is taking or receiving, and advise the client of these interactions.
   i   A health care worker must provide health services in a manner that is culturally sensitive to the needs of his or her clients.

2   Health care workers to obtain consent

Prior to commencing a treatment or service, a health care worker must ensure that consent appropriate to that treatment or service has been obtained and complies with the laws of the jurisdiction.

3   Appropriate conduct in relation to treatment advice

1   A health care worker must accept the right of his or her clients to make informed choices in relation to their health care.

2 A health care worker must not attempt to dissuade a client from seeking or continuing medical treatment.

3 A health care worker must communicate and co-operate with colleagues and other health service providers and agencies in the best interests of their clients.

4 *Health care workers to report concerns about the conduct of other health care workers*

A health care worker who, in the course of providing treatment or care, forms the reasonable belief that another health care worker has placed or is placing clients at serious risk of harm must refer the matter to the Health Ombudsman.

5 *Health care workers to take appropriate action in response to adverse events*

1 A health care worker must take appropriate and timely measures to minimise harm to clients when an adverse event occurs in the course of providing treatment or care.

2 Without limiting subclause (1), a health care worker must:

   a ensure that appropriate first aid is available to deal with any adverse event
   b obtain appropriate emergency assistance in the event of any serious adverse event
   c promptly disclose the adverse event to the client and take appropriate remedial steps to reduce the risk of recurrence
   d report the adverse event to the relevant authority, where appropriate.

6 *Health care workers to adopt standard precautions for infection control*

1 A health care worker must adopt standard precautions for the control of infection in the course of providing treatment or care.

2 Without limiting subclause (1), a health care worker who carries out skin penetration or other invasive procedure must comply with the *Public Health Act 2005* (Qld) under which such procedures are regulated.

7 *Health care workers diagnosed with infectious medical conditions*

1 A health care worker who has been diagnosed with a medical condition that can be passed on to clients must ensure that he or she practises in a manner that does not put clients at risk.

2 Without limiting subclause (1), a health care worker who has been diagnosed with a medical condition that can be passed on to clients must take and follow advice from a suitably qualified registered health practitioner on the necessary steps to be taken to modify his or her practice to avoid the possibility of transmitting that condition to clients.

8 *Health care workers not to make claims to cure certain serious illnesses*

1 A health care worker must not claim or represent that he or she is qualified, able or willing to cure cancer or other terminal illnesses.

2 A health care worker who claims to be able to treat or alleviate the symptoms of cancer or other terminal illnesses must be able to substantiate such claims.

9 Health care workers not to misinform their clients

1 A health care worker must not engage in any form of misinformation or misrepresentation in relation to the products or services he or she provides or the qualifications, training or professional affiliations he or she holds.

2 Without limiting subclause (1):

   a   a health care worker must not use his or her possession of a particular qualification to mislead or deceive clients or the public as to his or her competence in a field of practice or ability to provide treatment

   b   a health care worker must provide truthful information as to his or her qualifications, training or professional affiliations

   c   a health care worker must not make claims either directly to clients or in advertising or promotional materials about the efficacy of treatment or services he or she provides if those claims cannot be substantiated.

*10 Health care workers not to practise under the influence of alcohol
or unlawful substances*

1 A health care worker must not provide treatment or care to clients while under the influence of alcohol or unlawful substances.

2 A health care worker who is taking prescribed medication must obtain advice from the prescribing health practitioner or dispensing pharmacist on the impact of the medication on his or her ability to practise and must refrain from treating or caring for clients in circumstances where his or her capacity is or may be impaired.

11 Health care workers with certain mental or physical impairment

1 A health care worker must not provide treatment or care to clients while suffering from a physical or mental impairment, disability, condition or disorder (including an addiction to alcohol or a drug, whether or not prescribed) that places or is likely to place clients at risk of harm.

2 Without limiting subclause (1), if a health care worker has a mental or physical impairment that could place clients at risk, the health care worker must seek advice from a suitably qualified health practitioner to determine whether, and in what ways, he or she should modify his or her practice, including stopping practice if necessary.

12 Health care workers not to financially exploit clients

1 A health care worker must not financially exploit their clients.

2 Without limiting subclause (1):

   a   a health care worker must only provide services or treatments to clients that are designed to maintain or improve clients' health or wellbeing

   b   a health care worker must not accept or offer financial inducements or gifts as a part of client referral arrangements with other health care workers

   c   a health care worker must not ask clients to give, lend or bequeath money or gifts that will benefit the health care worker directly or indirectly.

13 Health care workers not to engage in sexual misconduct

1 A health care worker must not engage in behaviour of a sexual or close personal nature with a client.
2 A health care worker must not engage in a sexual or other inappropriate close personal, physical or emotional relationship with a client.
3 A health care worker should ensure that a reasonable period of time has elapsed since the conclusion of the therapeutic relationship before engaging in a sexual relationship with a client.

14 Health care workers to comply with relevant privacy laws

A health care worker must comply with the relevant privacy laws that apply to clients' health information, including the *Privacy Act 1988* (Cth) and the *Information Privacy Act 2009* (Qld).

15 Health care workers to keep appropriate records

1 A health care worker must maintain accurate, legible and up-to-date clinical records for each client consultation and ensure that these are held securely and not subject to unauthorised access.
2 A health care worker must take necessary steps to facilitate clients' access to information contained in their health records if requested.
3 A health care worker must facilitate the transfer of a client's health record in a timely manner when requested to do so by the client or their legal representative.

16 Health care workers to be covered by appropriate insurance

A health care worker should ensure that appropriate indemnity insurance arrangements are in place in relation to his or her practice.

17 Health care workers to display code and other information

1 A health care worker must display or make available a copy of each of the following documents at all premises where the health care worker carries on his or her practice:

a a copy of this Code of Conduct
b a document that gives information about the way in which clients may make a complaint to the Health Ombudsman.

2 Copies of these documents must be displayed or made available in a manner that makes them easily visible or accessible to clients.
3 This clause does not apply to any of the following premises:

1 the premises of any entity within the public health system as defined in the *Hospital and Health Boards Act 2011*
2 private health facilities as defined in the *Private Health Facilities Act 1999*

3   premises of the Queensland Ambulance Service as defined in the *Ambulance Service Act 1991*

4   premises of approved aged care service providers within the meaning of the *Aged Care Act 1997* (Cth).

Significantly there is now provision for collaboration between Queensland, Victoria, South Australia and New South Wales to allow for the enforcement of prohibition remedies even when the person involved has moved interstate or is working interstate.[35]

Notes

1   Refer to s 113 of the National Law.
2   *Health Practitioner Regulation National Law Act 2009* (Qld); *Health Practitioner Regulation National Law (NSW) Act 2009*; *Health Practitioner Regulation National Law (Victoria) Act 2009*; *Health Practitioner Regulation National Law (South Australia) Act 2010*; *Health Practitioner Regulation National Law (WA) Act 2010*; *Health Practitioner Regulation National Law (Tasmania) Act 2010*; *Health Practitioner Regulation (National Uniform Legislation) Act 2010* (NT); *Health Practitioner Regulation National Law (ACT) Act 2010*.
3   *Health Practitioner Regulation National Law Act 2009* s 7A–7C.
4   Section 115.
5   Sections 116 and 118.
6   *Health Practitioner Regulation National Law Act 2009* s 113.
7   *Penev v County Court (Vic) [2013] VSC 143*.
8   *Penev v County Court (Vic) [2013] VSC 143, [4]–[6]*.
9   *Penev v County Court (Vic) [2013] VSC 143, [54]*.
10   M. Weir, 'Holding Out and Protected Titles—Issues for Non-registrant Complementary and Alternative Health Practitioners', 25 (2018) *Journal of Law and Medicine* 4, 1033–1041. 1040.
11   Ibid., 1041.
12   Ibid., 1041.
13   Ibid., 1041.
14   Ibid., 1041.
15   S. Janz & J. Adams, 'Acupuncture by Another Name: Dry Needling in Australia', 6 (2011) *Australian Journal of Acupuncture and Chinese Medicine*, 3–11; James Dunning et al., 'Dry Needling: A Literature Review with Implications for Clinical Practice Guidelines', (2014) 19 *Phys Ther Rev* 4, 252–65.
16   *Health Practitioner Regulation National Law Act 2009*, s 121.
17   Ibid., s 122.
18   Ibid., s 123.
19   R.L. Drake, A.W. Vogl & M. Mitchell, *Gray's Anatomy for Students*, 2nd ed., Churchill Livingstone, New York, 2010, p. 58.
20   [2004] SADC 190 (22 December 2004).
21   Ibid., para. 66.
22   Ibid., para. 66.
23   Ibid., para. 68.
24   https://www.health.govt.nz/our-work/regulation-health-and-disability-system/health-practitioners-competence-assurance-act (accessed 18 September 2021).
25   https://www.health.govt.nz/our-work/regulation-health-and-disability-system/health-practitioners-competence-assurance-act/restricted-activities-under-act (accessed 18 February 2022).
26   Osteopathic Council New Zealand, *Osteopathic Scope of Practice Reform*, Wellington, 2010.

27 https://www.health.govt.nz/our-work/regulation-health-and-disability-system/health-practitioners-competence-assurance-act/restricted-activities-under-act

28 https://www.health.govt.nz/our-work/regulation-health-and-disability-system/health-practitioners-competence-assurance-act/restricted-activities-under-act

29 www.health.nsw.gov.au/phact/Documents/Code_of_Conduct_unregistered_health_practitioners_-_poster_-_2012_Regulation.pdf (accessed 10 September 2021).

30 www.coaghealthcouncil.gov.au/Announcements/ArtMID/527/ArticleID/54/Final-Report-A-National-Code-of-Conduct-for-health-care-workers (accessed 10 October 2021) COAG Final Report, p. 55.

31 https://www.healthcomplaints.tas.gov.au/national-code-of-conduct (accessed 10 October 2021).

32 Note to clause 5 the *Public Health Act 2010* defines skin penetration procedure as any procedure (whether medical or not) that involves skin penetration (such as acupuncture, tattooing, ear piercing or hair removal), and includes any procedure declared by the regulations to be a skin penetration procedure, but does not include: (a) any procedure carried out by a registered health practitioner, or by a person acting under the direction or supervision of a registered health practitioner, in the course of providing a health service; or (b) any procedure declared by the regulations not to be a skin penetration procedure.

33 *Health Complaints Act 2016* s 3. (Vic).

34 Refer to s 7 *Health Ombudsman Act 2013* (Qld) and s 4 *Health and Community Services Complaints Act 2004* (SA) NSW Code of Conduct.

35 Refer to *Health and Community Services Complaints Act 2004* (SA) s 56 EA; *Health Care Complaints Act 1993* s 41 AA and *Public Health Regulation 2012* (NSW) s 93A; *Health Complaints Act 2016* (Vic) s 102; *Health Ombudsman Act 2013* s 77 (Qld) and Regulation 3 and 4.

5 Negligence and professional responsibilities

Everyone has the responsibility to avoid causing injury to other persons or their property. This obligation applies to virtually any activity, from driving a motor vehicle to providing professional advice or treatment. This principle of law was expressed in the famous case of *Donoghue v Stevenson*,[1] where Lord Atkin stated: 'You must take reasonable care to avoid acts or omissions which you can reasonably foresee would be likely to injure your neighbour.' To breach this obligation is described as 'negligence', or a 'negligent act'.

This principle of law applies to all professional people in the course of their professional activities. For example, medical doctors, complementary medicine practitioners, lawyers and engineers all have an obligation to take reasonable care in their practice to avoid acts or omissions that are likely to injure a client, whether physically or financially.

Negligence has been defined as 'the omission to do something which a reasonable man, guided on those considerations which ordinarily regulate the conduct of human affairs would do, or doing something which a prudent or reasonable man would not do'.[2] Attention is focused on whether the conduct fell below the required standard. It is unnecessary to show that the person who did the act or omission had a particular state of mind or intention.

This chapter will discuss the liability of practitioners for negligence and how they can both protect against professional malpractice claims and improve the professionalism of the service they provide. As part of the practitioner's duty, the obligation to obtain consent to treatment and to warn of the risks of treatment will be discussed. This chapter also deals with the mechanism for complaints against practitioners under the health rights complaints legislation that applies in all states and territories.

BOX 5.1

Action plan

- Provide a standard of care to your clients appropriate to a reasonably competent member of your profession.
- Be aware that a duty of care may arise even through a phone call or social occasion.
- Follow up referrals made by you in your practice.
- Keep up to date with developments in your profession.

DOI: 10.4324/9781003195931-5

- Provide clients with good information about treatment and warn them of the risks of treatment.
- Obtain consent to treatment from clients.
- Understand your entitlements and obligations under relevant health rights complaints legislation.

Complementary medicine and negligence

Complementary medicine treatment generates few adverse outcomes compared with orthodox medicine, because of the nature of the modalities and philosophy. There is, however, potential for serious and even fatal outcomes from complementary medicine, and this requires practitioners to consider their professional responsibilities carefully. Every state and territory in Australia has passed civil liability legislation that describes the principles of liability in negligence of a professional person and other matters that impact on the ability to mount an action and to claim recovery for personal injury claims.[3] These statutes, called here 'the civil liability legislation', are similar between the states but not identical. As these statutes are complex it is not possible to give a detailed commentary on these provisions in this book. Rather, an outline of some important provisions is included.

Negligence claims against complementary medicine practitioners

In Australia, the United Kingdom and New Zealand, there are limited numbers of reported cases of negligence actions against complementary medicine practitioners.
  The reasons for this record might be:

- *Better communication.* Negligence actions tend to arise in a therapeutic environment when the client–practitioner relationship has broken down and communication has failed or has been insufficient. Complementary medicine generally emphasises synergistic, client-centred healing, with a focus on communication between the practitioner and client.[4] This type of therapeutic relationship will often avoid the misunderstandings that provide the basis of many negligence actions. Where communication is open and responsibility for the therapeutic outcome is shared, unsuccessful treatment will be less likely to focus the client on any shortcomings of the practitioner.
- *Less intrusive.* Complementary medicine is by nature less intrusive and interventionist than orthodox medicine, which often relies on surgical procedures and prescribing potentially harmful drugs. There is simply less scope for injury in most forms of treatment undertaken by complementary medicine practitioners.
- *Less reporting of adverse outcomes.* A stigma may attach to attending complementary medicine practitioners, which may dissuade clients from complaining of negligence and thereby exposing their use of such services.[5] This tendency may decrease as complementary medicine becomes more widely accepted.
- *No professional indemnity insurance.* There is little point in suing someone who is not covered by professional indemnity insurance unless that person has substantial assets to satisfy a judgement. Some complementary medicine practitioners do not have indemnity insurance, which is a disincentive to litigation.[6]
- *Difficulty in establishing standard.* It may be difficult to determine the appropriate level of competence required by a practitioner, as some modalities defy scientific

explanation and measurement. In addition, many modalities rely on individual treatments for a particular client at a particular time. This makes it difficult to apply the appropriate test of negligence against which to measure the competence of the practitioner.[7] There are few agreed competency standards for complementary medicine modalities.[8] It is more difficult to determine negligence when there is no agreement on what are expected or required standards in practice or what treatment outcome can be expected for a particular illness, condition or client.

- *Monetary value of claim.* The monetary value of the claims likely to result from complementary medicine would encourage parties to settle before any court hearing. This leaves no public record of the claim.
- *Less serious conditions treated.* Complementary medicine practitioners are more often involved in treating chronic, sub-acute or sub-clinical conditions that rarely involve the risky emergency treatment likely to generate negligence claims.

Despite these disincentives to litigation, the number of actions brought against complementary practitioners may increase. This may occur as the number of visits to complementary medicine practitioners increases and there is greater incorporation of complementary medicine within formal health structures as more complementary medicine practitioners are acknowledged as registered health practitioners.

Injury caused by complementary medicine

There is relevant case law in Australia, to indicate that the use of complementary medicine does sometimes result in injury or harm including death. Bensoussan and Myers[9] have recounted examples of injury to patients of traditional Chinese medicine based on adverse herbal reactions, misdiagnosis, failure to refer, failure to explain precautions, poisoning and adverse interactions with pharmaceuticals.[10] Bensoussan and Myers have suggested that traditional Chinese medicine practitioners experience a client-adverse event once every eight months, from consumption of substances causing toxicity to allergic reactions, infection, physical injury, convulsions and fainting.[11]

Also described are risks associated with acupuncture,[12] including local and systemic infection, and trauma such as nerve damage, burns and severe bruising. Despite these incidents, Bensoussan and Myers conclude: 'It is highly unlikely that the practice of TCM [traditional Chinese medicine] poses as great a risk to public safety as the practice of western medicine.'[13] There is a substantial body of literature and cases about adverse events in chiropractic and osteopathy.[14] One study found 78 significant incidents from 1934 to 1992, excluding those incidents where there was complete or near recovery or an unknown outcome.[15]

Codes of Conduct for Unregistered Health Workers in a number of States contain examples of negative outcomes from the activities of both registered and unregistered complementary medicine practitioners, which provide guidance about what is not acceptable professional practice.[16]

Lack of authority

The lack of case law relevant to the negligence of complementary medicine practitioners in the United Kingdom, Australia and New Zealand means there is no well-developed set of legal principles that can be applied to determine the appropriate standard of care for complementary medicine practitioners. For this reason, reference to case law that is relevant to the negligence of medical doctors will be applied by analogy to complementary medicine practitioners, then a discussion of the reported cases of claims for negligence involving complementary medicine practitioners will follow.

There is some useful case law in the United States, where many issues relevant to complementary medicine have been litigated. The principles of law discussed in these cases provide some assistance about the possible issues and conclusions in this country.

General principles of negligence

The law relating to negligence seeks to compensate a party who has suffered an injury because of negligent conduct. The law asks:

* Did a duty of care exist?
* Has this duty been breached?
* Was the injury caused by the act in question?
* Has damage been suffered?

Duty of care

A duty of care exists when the relationship between the parties warrants the imposition on one party of an obligation of care for the benefit of the other. The law asks whether the person in question should have had the other person within their contemplation as possibly being injured by their negligent act. Healthcare professionals do not owe a duty of care to the world at large. It is necessary to establish some type of legal relationship between the plaintiff and defendant.[17]

The establishment of the duty of care is particularly important where the link between a person doing an act and a person injured is tenuous—for example, where a builder builds a house negligently and the local authority certifies that work. If the building deteriorates because of that shoddy work, is the local authority liable to the house owner?

In most situations involving complementary medicine practitioners, there is no difficulty in establishing the existence of a duty of care. It is virtually assumed to exist in most cases about medical practitioners.[18]

It is normally a simple task to demonstrate that, if negligent treatment or advice is provided by a complementary medicine practitioner, it is reasonably foreseeable that injury could occur to a client. There is no doubt that the law implies an obligation on that therapist to use care, diligence and skill in the treatment and advice given.

BOX 5.2

Practice tip: Situations when a duty of care may arise

A duty of care may arise unexpectedly for the practitioner in the following situations:

* An informal social setting. At a party on Saturday evening, someone you have never met before asks you about back pain referred down his arm. As you are a

chiropractor, you proffer the view that it sounds like a minor subluxation and noth-ing serious, but say you would be happy to see him the following week. The pain was in fact the warnings of a heart attack that the patient suffered on the Sunday. An argument could be mounted that your advice indicated that you undertook to take this person as a client and a duty of care arose, even in that informal situation. This suggests the need to avoid giving professional opinions in a social situation without proper examination. Advise the client to seek professional assistance if the problem worsens.

- A telephone conversation. Advice given on the telephone may create a duty of care where a client relates symptoms and the practitioner attempts to analyse or diag-nose the problem and suggests treatment. Don't give advice over the phone or do so with a full understanding of the potential for liability without proper examination.
- Treatment of friends or family. If you are treating friends or relatives, approach their care as you would that of any other person. You should open a patient card and follow all the usual proper procedures fully. With friends or relatives, there may be a tendency to relax and not provide the same standard of care. A duty of care will arise.

Breach of duty of care

If a duty of care exists, has a breach of duty occurred?

General test

As people are involved in myriad activities, it is impossible to specify required rules of conduct for every circumstance. The law therefore applies the standard of a 'reasona-ble person' to provide a model of what conduct is required to satisfy a duty of care.[19] In an everyday activity such as driving a car, the question of whether you have attained the required standard will be judged on what a reasonable person would have done in that situation. For professionals such as complementary medicine practitioners, the standard required is generally the proficiency of a reasonably competent member of that profession.

Reasonable person test in relation to medical practitioners

It is worthwhile to briefly consider the negligence liability of medical practitioners. For many modalities, this is the area of practice most closely aligned with comple-mentary medicine.

General duty

This relevant test for a medical practitioner is described by McNair J in *Bolam v Friern Hospital Management Committee*:[20]

The test is the standard of the ordinary skilled man exercising and professing to have that special skill. A man need not possess the highest expert skill at the risk of being found negligent. It is a well-established law that it is sufficient if he exercises the ordinary skill of an ordinary competent man exercising that particular art.

The High Court of Australia confirmed in *Rogers v Whitaker*[21] that:

> The law imposes on a medical practitioner a duty to exercise reasonable care and skill in the provision of professional advice and treatment. The duty is a 'single comprehensive duty covering all the ways in which a doctor is called upon to exercise his skill and judgement'. It extends to the examination, diagnosis and treatment of the patient and the provision of information in an appropriate case.

Specialists

The content of the standard of care can vary if the doctor professes to have a particular skill or speciality. The High Court in *Rogers v Whitaker* stated that, for specialists:

> The standard of reasonable care and skill required is that of the ordinary skilled person exercising and professing to have that special skill, in this case the skill of an ophthalmic surgeon specialising in corneal and anterior segment surgery.[22]

It was necessary in that case to apply an appropriate test based on the particular and quite narrow speciality of the doctor involved. It would have been inappropriate to apply a test relevant to a general surgeon or a general practitioner. Thus the particular knowledge and expertise of an individual will impact on the standard expected where it can be shown that a practitioner holds him or herself out as having an acknowledged speciality.[23]

For a general practitioner, the standard would be that of a reasonably competent general practitioner. A specialist standard of care for a complementary medicine practitioner might be applied if it could be shown they profess to have the additional training and experience to undertake a higher level of practice. For example, an osteopath might hold him or herself out as having a speciality in relation to manipulations of the cranium. The chiropractic profession acknowledges some chiropractors as having practice specialities. This might allow the imposition of a higher standard of care in relation to those types of procedures. A naturopath might be deemed to specialise in treating chronic fatigue syndrome based on a differential fee structure, professional acknowledgement, advertising and promotional activities of the practitioner.

BOX 5.3

Practice tip

When advertising particular skills in 'difficult cases' or in relation to specified maladies such as sports injuries, the possible implication of a higher standard of care should be considered. In litigation, the defendant may seek to cast doubt on your expertise to treat specific diseases and the basis for the claims made in advertising. Holding out or advertising yourself as specially qualified or experienced may provide the basis for the imposition of the higher 'specialist' standard of care in relation to your procedures and advice.[24]

Beginners

Although there is clearly a need to provide 'on-the-job' training for inexperienced professionals, the law generally favours a policy of securing compensation for victims of negligence. Accordingly, professionals are expected to attain the competence of a person reasonably skilled and proficient in the calling.[25]

Practitioners cannot escape liability by arguing that the standard of care should be lower because of their inexperience. The law will impose on them a minimum standard of performance below which they must not fall. Inexperience is not an excuse. This should focus complementary medicine practitioners on the need for practical training, continuing education and, in some circumstances, proper supervision by a more experienced practitioner.

Approved professional practice

The determination of whether negligence has occurred is based on whether the act was what could be expected of a reasonably competent practitioner.[26] If the act was in accordance with accepted practices of the profession, this will assist in showing that negligence did not occur. Conformity with standard practice will usually (but not always) dispel negligence, as it indicates that the defendant has acted as other professionals in the field would have done.[27]

Failure to comply with standard procedures is a strong indication of negligence, especially if the injury caused was the injury that the standard procedure is intended to avoid. In this situation, the onus of proof to prove there was no negligence may switch to the defendant practitioner.[28]

In England, the courts have accepted, based on *Bolam*'s case, that the standard of care of a doctor is a matter of medical judgement and will respect a therapeutic approach that is based on a responsible body of professional opinion. The court is loath to impose its own standard, especially when dealing with a matter relevant to diagnosis and treatment. The High Court in *Rogers v Whitaker* has stated in relation to diagnosis and treatment that the *Bolam* principle has not always been applied. Although professional standards and procedures are important, the 'standard is not determined solely or even primarily by reference to the practice followed or supported by a responsible body of opinion in the relevant profession or trade'.[29] Rather, the court is the ultimate determinant of what is or is not negligent activity. This is the Australian 'common law' approach to professional negligence.

This was a factor in the Victorian Court of Appeal decision of *Forder v Hutchinson*,[30] where the court concluded that the standard of care to be applied in relation to the defendant naturopath/osteopath was not based entirely upon the standards of the profession. In that case, the court noted the *Bolam* principle was not always applied.

Statutory duty of care

The common law approach has now been varied by the civil liability legislation in each jurisdiction of Australia, which provides that if 'professionals' follow procedures deemed acceptable by their profession (even if there may be different views on the matter and the activity is not universally accepted), they will be deemed not to be in breach of their duty. This applies as long as those procedures are not 'irrational'.

This test applies a varied *Bolam* test to the duty of care. The test will place greater emphasis on professional opinion to determine negligence as against the common law principles described in *Rogers v Whitaker* that preserved for the court the ultimate decision of what was or was not competent practice. In many cases, it is suggested that the result of a claim will not be changed by the application of the statutory test.

An example of this provision is section 5O of the *Civil Liability Act 2002* (NSW), which provides:

1 A person practising a profession ('a professional') does not incur a liability in negligence arising from the provision of a professional service if it is established that the professional acted in a manner that (at the time the service was provided) was widely accepted in Australia by peer professional opinion as competent professional practice.
2 However, peer professional opinion cannot be relied on for the purposes of this section if the court considers that the opinion is irrational.
3 The fact that there are differing peer professional opinions widely accepted in Australia concerning a matter does not prevent any one or more (or all) of those opinions being relied on for the purposes of this section.
4 Peer professional opinion does not have to be universally accepted to be considered widely accepted.

One issue that may be addressed by a court is whether a complementary medicine practitioner qualifies as a 'professional' within the terms of the statute.[31] The New South Wales Supreme Court decision of *Zhang v Hardas* involved an action for negligence by a chiropractor and the question was whether a chiropractor was a professional. It was acknowledged that:

Section 5O of the Civil Liability Act does not define 'profession'. However, it was enacted in a context in which (a) it was plain that the conventional medical profession was squarely within the mischief to which it was directed and (b) legislation treated chiropractors in ways which were similar to medical practitioners. The Chiropractors Tribunal operated similarly to the Medical Tribunal, especially insofar as provision was made for regulation, involving statutory concepts of professional misconduct and unsatisfactory professional conduct. The relevant statute in 2007, the *Chiropractors Act 2001*, consistently treated chiropractors as professionals. There is every reason for the undefined term 'professional' in s 5O to extend to occupations regarded by the same Legislature as 'professional'.

The foregoing is sufficient to conclude that chiropractors were regarded, for the purposes of the *Civil Liability Act* in 2007, as practising a profession. It will also be seen that the notion of a licensed monopoly of people who practise spinal manipulation, with educational qualifications and mechanisms for admitting and excluding those who meet or fail to meet those standards, also appears to apply. It will also be plain from the legislative history that the same would not have been true some decades before.[32]

Although the comments in *Zhang v Hardas* are not fulsome in accepting that chiropractic and probably other registered complementary medicine modalities satisfy the definition of 'professional' it is suggested that some complementary medicine practitioners may qualify as a 'professional' under this legislation, based upon:

*   the registered status of practitioners of Chinese medicine, osteopathy and chiropractic
*   the level of education of many complementary medicine practitioners in Australia (at tertiary level for osteopaths, chiropractors and Chinese medicine practitioners, and for a number of other modalities such as naturopaths, with movement towards requiring degree-level training for many modalities)
*   their status in health complaints legislation in all states; their acknowledgement in the Commonwealth *Therapeutic Goods Act* and state and Commonwealth privacy legislation
*   the membership by many practitioners of professional associations, and their obligation to adhere to a professional association code of ethics, and
*   the establishment of many pan- and multi-professional national professional associations such as the Australian Natural Therapists Association, the Australian Traditional Medicine Society, Massage Australia and the National Naturopaths and Herbalists Association of Australia.

Those who do not qualify would be subject to the above described common law principles.

This issue has particular importance for complementary medicine practitioners, as in some situations the accepted professional practice may be difficult to ascertain. There is a distinct lack of settled protocols and procedures, which makes the task of ascertaining accepted professional practice more difficult. Increasingly, modalities are adopting competency standards that may provide some guidance for a court when it is assessing professional behaviour.

Misadventure

An unexpected result from treatment may not be the result of negligence, but may simply be a misadventure as the practitioner has acted in accordance with accepted professional practice: 'The law does not seek to punish all mistakes, only negligent mistakes.'[33]

An example is the authority of *Dwan v Farquhar and Ors*,[34] where a patient was infected with HIV after knee surgery. At the time, there was no means to screen blood for HIV, and there was no evidence to suggest that a surgeon would have advised on the risk of acquiring HIV from transfused blood. There was clearly an injury to the patient but, based on the medical knowledge at the time, there was no negligence by the medical practitioner.

Another example is the South Australian authority *Bawden v Marin*.[35] The authority is significant, as it is one of the very few reported cases outside the United States that relates to the negligence of a chiropractor. Here, an action for negligence was brought against a chiropractor for injuries sustained (broken ribs) during spinal manipulation. The court held for the chiropractor and concluded the plaintiff did suffer an injury that ought not to have been suffered, but that the injury was caused by misadventure. The court concluded that there was no evidence the chiropractor's treatment regime had fallen below the required standard of care for a chiropractor.

The court was saying that the broken ribs did occur as a result of the practitioner's acts, but the practitioner did not act negligently so there was no liability for that injury. This decision is discussed in more detail below.

How is the standard of care proven?

The plaintiff is obliged to demonstrate that, on the balance of probabilities, the practitioner has failed to attain the required standard of care. Proof of this will rely to a considerable extent on expert witnesses.

Normally, both the plaintiff and defendant will provide their own expert witnesses. An expert witness should reflect the modality under consideration, as this is the best means to gauge professional practice standards.[36] Thus a chiropractor should give evidence in regard to a claim made against a chiropractor, and a naturopath should give evidence in relation to a claim against a naturopath.

The level of deference given to expert evidence by medical practitioners in medical negligence cases is based to some extent on an acknowledgement by the court that many aspects of orthodox medicine have a proven scientific basis. Complementary medicine often does not reflect a scientific approach to healing; instead, it relies on intuitive, anecdotal or traditional evidence. The legal system is fundamentally conservative in nature.[37] In considering the appropriate standard of care of complementary medicine practitioners, a court may be more likely to make its own assessment of what should be the practice of a particular modality. This would apply more forcefully the further away from the accepted and well-regulated professions one gets. When dealing with complementary medicine, a court may consider an activity that the profession may consider appropriate to be negligent.

Pursuant to the civil liability legislation discussed above, a court could conceivably deem as 'irrational', and thereby not within the protection of that legislation, an act conforming with standard professional practice of a complementary medicine modality if that practice is not supported by acceptable scientific evidence. Although we await the judicial interpretation of these provisions, an overly broad interpretation of the term 'irrational' would risk damage to the statutory objectives of this legislation.

The civil liability legislation applies the varied *Bolam* approach to the liability of health professionals that places emphasis on the profession's view of appropriate practice. This would override the stricter *Rogers v Whitaker* approach, which suggested that the court was the final arbiter of what was or was not a negligent act or omission. For practitioners who do not qualify as a 'professional', the stricter *Rogers v Whitaker* approach would still apply.

BOX 5.4

Practice tip

Whenever you are contemplating controversial or fringe techniques at the edge of accepted professional practice, consider how a conservative court, in reviewing your treatment, may view this approach.

Causation

Once the plaintiff has established that a duty of care has arisen and has been breached, it is necessary for the plaintiff to show that, on the balance of probabilities, the breach of care caused the damage that was suffered. This relies on a common sense assessment of the connection between the negligent act and the damage suffered.[38] The question is whether a particular act or omission can fairly and properly be considered a cause of the damage suffered.[39] If there is evidence that, despite the negligent act, the damage would have occurred anyway, there is no causation and no liability.

For example, a client may present with stomach pain. A practitioner misdiagnoses the symptoms as indigestion when the actual cause of the pain is poisoning. If the client dies, an important issue of causation is whether the client would have died of poisoning in any event. If it could be shown that, given the type or amount of poison ingested, the client was doomed to die, then there would be no causal connection between the negligent diagnosis and the damage suffered. It would not have mattered if the correct diagnosis had been made, because the damage would have been suffered anyway.

The civil liability legislation now places a greater burden on the plaintiff to indicate a factual connection between the alleged negligence and the injury said to have been suffered in that case. These provisions require it to be shown that a breach of duty was a necessary condition of the occurrence of the harm. Examples of these provisions are found in section 11 of the *Civil Liability Act 2003* (Qld) and section 39 of the *Civil Liability Act 1936* (SA).

The legislation also asks the court to consider the appropriateness of extending liability for the negligence in that case. This adds an element of public policy into these considerations, which may tend to limit the liability of practitioners in some situations. These provisions also provide that a person is not liable in negligence for harm suffered as a result of the materialisation of an inherent risk—that is, the risk of something occurring that cannot be avoided by the exercise of reasonable care and skill. Examples of these provisions are found in section 34 of the *Civil Liability Act 1936* (SA) and section 5I of the *Civil Liability Act 2002* (NSW).

Thus, if a practitioner acts competently but an inherent risk of treatment eventuates, then the practitioner may not be liable for that injury subject to comments below about the requirement to warn of inherent risks of treatment prior to the client consenting to the procedure.

Causation was a factor considered in the Victorian Court of Appeal case of *Forder v Hutchinson*,[40] where a claim was made in regard to a neck manipulation performed by an osteopath/naturopath. Expert evidence suggested the manipulation could have caused the injury of which the plaintiff complained. The court considered that even if expert medical evidence suggests no more than an event is capable of being the cause of an observable medical condition, it might be possible to infer, based on the totality of the evidence, that it was a cause of that condition.

BOX 5.5

Practice tip

A naturopath is treating a client for persistent headaches. This naturopath may not ascertain that the client has a brain tumour. To establish liability for negligence, a number of things would need to be proven on the balance of probabilities:

- that the naturopath had a duty to diagnose medical conditions
- if the client was advised to see a doctor, that he or she would have done so
- if the client had seen a doctor, that the correct diagnosis would have been made, and
- that the correct treatment would have been given and the damage would have been averted—that is, that the tumour was not already inoperable.[41]

Causation may be clear where there is a poisoning by adulterated herbs, burning from moxibustion (a traditional Chinese medicine technique that involves the burning [often close to the body of the client] of mugwort, a small, spongy herb, to facilitate healing) or a fracture caused by a chiropractic manipulation, but it may be more problematic when there could be many reasons for a particular injury. A client may undergo treatment by a practitioner and become sick shortly afterwards. Liability would only attach if the plaintiff could demonstrate that the treatment by that practitioner caused the sickness. If there is no established link between the treatment and the sickness or injury, there may be no causation. This evidence may not be readily available, and may in some cases provide a barrier to a client's recovering damages for negligence.

Kirby J, in *Chappel v Hart*,[42] provided a list of possible reasons to displace a finding of causation in relation to an event, including:

- that the damage was coincidental and not related to the breach
- that the damage was inevitable and would have occurred even without the breach, and
- that the event was the result of unreasonable action by the plaintiff.

Susceptible plaintiffs

What if a practitioner injures a client who is inherently susceptible (for example, a person who has an allergic reaction to royal jelly or massage oil, or has soft bones) where no injury would have occurred to a person of normal physiology? If the practitioner has acted as a reasonably competent practitioner would have, there may be no liability for that damage. This would involve a consideration of what steps, investigations and examinations would have been reasonable for the practitioner to do to protect against known potential adverse reactions or susceptibilities. If it was reasonable to take certain steps to avoid potential negative reactions, the susceptibility may not excuse the practitioner. If the client knew of their susceptibility and failed to reveal it on being questioned, this might create grounds for contributory negligence (where the plaintiff has contributed to the injury by his or her own negligence). This might reduce the liability of the practitioner or even excuse the practitioner entirely.

Once it is demonstrated that some trauma was foreseeable from the initial negligent act, liability will attach to any unexpected damages that might ensue. For example, if an acupuncturist causes a minor infection through negligence and, because of the client's inherent susceptibility, this results in systemic septicaemia, then this would be an event covered by the original negligent act.[43]

Follow-up

A New South Wales case indicates that liability could arise where a practitioner fails to follow up the treatment of a client and as a result the client suffers injury. In *Tai v Hatzistravou*,[44] a doctor was deemed liable for negligence due to not ensuring that a patient followed through with a curette operation that would have resulted in the discovery of cancer. As a result of the delay, the patient required a more radical procedure. The judge considered that the doctor had a duty to keep his opinion before the client so she could decide whether to proceed with the operation. This issue could arise for a complementary medicine practitioner who recommends referral to a medical doctor but does not follow up that recommendation and the client then suffers damage as a result.

Intervening act

An intervening act may destroy the connection between the negligent act and the damage suffered. Consider the case of an acupuncturist who negligently treats a client and causes slight injury. That client is taken to hospital where she is given negligent treatment and as a result suffers brain damage. This would not normally relieve the liability of the acupuncturist, as the possibility of negligent treatment by a third party is a reasonably foreseeable event. The acupuncturist may be liable for all the injuries suffered, including the injury caused by the hospital. If, however, the negligence of the hospital amounts to gross negligence, this may override any liability for the initial negligence by the acupuncturist, as gross negligence by a third party, such as a hospital, may not be reasonably foreseeable.

Onus of proof

A plaintiff will be required to demonstrate that a breach of duty has occurred, and damage has ensued as a result. Once this is established, the onus of proof does not shift, but the defendant may be obliged to show that the plaintiff should not recover damages.[45]

Damage

Once negligence and causation are established, if a plaintiff suffers damage, damages may be awarded. Damages cover such matters as:

* hospital, nursing and medical expenses
* loss of wages up to the trial
* loss of capacity for future earnings, and
* nervous shock.

The family of a deceased client may be entitled to the recovery of damages under statute.[46]

New Zealand provisions

New Zealand has comprehensive 'no-fault' compensation legislation, which may deal with claims against registered health practitioners. The *Accident Compensation Act 2001* provides for compensation to be payable in relation to 'treatment injury', which is personal injury suffered by a person seeking treatment from registered health professionals. If a claim is available under these provisions, it is a bar to a common law claim for compensation against the practitioner.

'Registered health professional' is defined regulation 7 of the *Accident Compensation (Definitions) Regulations* 2019 as including only orthodox medicine practitioners—for example, medical practitioners, physiotherapists as well as osteopaths and chiropractors. This suggests that, other than for a claim for negligence against a chiropractor or an osteopath, a claimant for injury from an act of another complementary medicine practitioner would be obliged to commence a common law action in tort or in contract, generally along the same lines as discussed above and below.

Application to complementary medicine

Although the authorities applicable to medical practitioners provide guidance, the fit between the law of negligence and complementary medicine is somewhat awkward.[47] Stone and Matthews argue that it is difficult to apply rational legal principles to intuitive and holistic healthcare therapies, as it may be difficult to show the necessary legal responsibility for a therapy that relies on patient responsibility and the practitioner's intuitive abilities, which may defy scientific explanation.[48]

What is likely to be the appropriate test of the standard of care? Authorities in Australia, the United States and Canada suggest that the standard of care for a complementary medicine practitioner is the same test that applies to professionals generally, and to medical practitioners in particular—that is, whether the practitioner has satisfied the standard of care for a reasonably competent complementary medicine practitioner.[49] As discussed in Australia under the principles discussed in *Rogers v Whitaker*, the High Court has maintained that it is not appropriate to rely only on professional practice to determine this test.

If a complementary medicine practitioner is deemed a 'professional', then the slightly different statutory duty of care under the civil liability legislation will be applied as discussed above—that is, a standard of care based on peer opinion. It is still worthwhile to consider relevant case law to understand how a court might approach applying the common law or statutory duty of care to a factual situation. A complementary medicine practitioner deemed not to be a 'professional' would be subject to the common law principles discussed in these cases that do not rely on the statutory duty of care.

Bawden v Marin

One of the few reported cases in Australia that deals with the liability of a complementary medicine practitioner is the South Australian Supreme Court Full Court decision in *Bawden v Marin*.[50] The plaintiff sought damages for what was said to be negligent spinal manipulation by a chiropractor, causing broken ribs.

The primary issue on appeal was the finding by a lower court judge that, although he accepted that the defendant's treatment caused the broken ribs, he did not consider that the defendant had fallen short of the appropriate standard of care.

The court heard the evidence of a medical doctor on behalf of the plaintiff, who suggested that for a person of her age (the plaintiff's age is not mentioned) the treatment should not have been undertaken. The plaintiff also relied on the evidence of a chiropractor, who suggested that the defendant could have used a chiropractic device called an 'activator' to limit the amount of force used in the manipulation.[51] The court noted that the failure to use such a device was not outside the normal discretion relating to chiropractic practice, and there was in fact ample evidence that there was nothing unreasonable in the defendant's decision to not use the activator in that case. The crux of the judgement was that:

> there was a total absence of any evidence to suggest that on the case history as disclosed to the respondent, and having regard to the number of occasions upon which he had in fact treated her and many other patients in much the same way and without ill effects, that his treatment on the last occasion which caused injury was in the circumstances negligent or as the learned judge said, was in breach of his duty of care to her.[52]

The court concluded unanimously that this was a case of an injury occurring by misadventure, and there was no evidence to support the conclusion that the respondent's treatment failed to attain the appropriate standard of care.

The case is significant as the court preferred the evidence of a chiropractor to that of a medical practitioner, and it applied the test of competence appropriate to a chiropractor, not a medical practitioner. By admitting into testimony the evidence of the medical practitioner, the case also suggests that it is appropriate evidence in a case involving the liability of a chiropractor. This is similar to the approach taken in the United States, where medical evidence is available to deal with questions of liability where there is an overlap in expertise with the practice in question.[53] In *Bawden v Marin*, the court applied standard principles of negligence relevant to medical doctors to this factual situation.[54]

Shakoor v Situ

A significant case that involved the liability of a traditional Chinese medicine (TCM) practitioner for negligence is the English decision in *Shakoor v Situ*.[55] This authority confirmed that the law will apply the standard of care of a TCM practitioner rather than an orthodox medicine practitioner in determining liability for negligence by a TCM practitioner. This authority further suggests that a court, in applying this test, will require complementary medicine practitioners to acknowledge that they practise within a predominantly orthodox medicine context.

FACTS

Shakoor v Situ involved a claim by the widow of Abdul Shakoor, who died after receiving a course of Chinese herbal medicine from the defendant. She contended that his death was caused by the negligence of the defendant, thereby entitling her to claim for damages.

The defendant was trained in China in both traditional and orthodox medicine, and had been practising in the United Kingdom for a number of years. He was not a registered medical practitioner but was a member of a TCM professional association.

The client had consulted the defendant about multiple benign lipomata (fatty deposits below the skin). His general practitioner had previously told him that the only remedy for this condition was surgery. The defendant prescribed a decoction of twelve herbs to be taken on alternate days. After taking the herbs, the client became ill and eventually suffered from liver failure and died after a liver transplant.

CAUSATION

The issue of causation was not a matter of controversy in this case. Judge Bernard Livesley QC (Deputy Judge of the High Court) held that the injury to the deceased's liver and his death were caused by an idiosyncratic reaction to the herbal concoction that was extremely rare and could not have been predicted.

The plaintiff argued that the defendant should have performed a liver function test prior to commencing the treatment and monitored the client during the eighteen days during which the substance was being used. These assertions were considered by Livesley QC to not have any prospect of success as the prior liver test would likely not have shown any abnormality and the monitoring would not have been able to ascertain that damage was being done before it was too late.[56]

The judge summarised the case as follows:

> The case for the claimant must therefore stand and fall on the allegation that it was negligent of the defendant to prescribe the decoction; alternatively to do so without warning the deceased of the risk of the injury to which ingestion of the decoction would expose him.[57]

APPROPRIATE TEST RE NEGLIGENCE

The significant argument presented by the plaintiff in this case was that the defendant had held himself out as the equivalent of a general medical practitioner specialising in skin complaints and should be judged by the standard of a reasonably competent medical practitioner in that field in the United Kingdom. It was argued that on that test he should have known about the possibility of injury as medical journals such as the *Lancet* had warned of the known risk of liver damage and, in one case, of death involving the ingestion of similar herbal medicine. If this type of test was accepted, it could expose a complementary medicine practitioner to liability for negligence even if they were acting in accordance with the requirements of their profession and would subject their practice to an entirely foreign healing philosophy.

It was also argued from the orthodox medicine perspective that, as this concoction would have no prospect of curing or ameliorating the client's ailment on a cost/benefit analysis, it should never have been used. The plaintiff suggested that if a practitioner decided to use the concoction then it should have been preceded by a suitable warning, which the plaintiff maintained the client would have heeded—therefore refusing treatment.

The defendant contended that the appropriate test to be applied was that of a reasonably competent TCM practitioner. In addition, he argued that even if the test asserted by the plaintiff was applied, he was not negligent by that standard. The defendant also argued that, as the plaintiff had not provided evidence of appropriate professional practice from a TCM practitioner, it was not possible to make a finding of negligence against him.[58]

DUTY OF CARE

Livesey QC accepted that the defendant had a duty to use reasonable care and not to cause harm. He noted that there was no authority in the common law system on the negligent liability of TCM practitioners. The judge accepted the defendant's argument in part by accepting that TCM practitioners should not be judged by the same standards as a medical doctor. This meant the standard of performance against which the defendant was to be judged was a reasonably competent TCM practitioner.

CONTENT OF DUTY OF CARE

The judge then discussed the content of the duty of a complementary medicine practitioner. He considered that there were three important points that needed to be made in the context of a practitioner prescribing a chemical or herbal remedy for internal consumption:[59]

1   A practitioner had to recognise that he or she is holding himself or herself out to practise within a system of law and medicine which will review the standard of care that has been taken in the care of a client.
2   Where a remedy is prescribed, it is not enough to say that the remedy is traditional and considered not harmful. It is the practitioner's duty to ensure that the remedy is actually not harmful or potentially harmful.
3   The practitioner must recognise the probability that any person suffering an adverse reaction to such a remedy is quite likely to find his or her way into an orthodox hospital and the incident may be written up in an orthodox medical journal. Such a practitioner should take steps to ascertain this evidence that could be satisfied by being a member of an association that searches the relevant literature and reports any relevant material to the practitioner.

The judge held that the defendant was not negligent as there was no possibility of predicting the adverse reaction to the treatment.

EVIDENCE RE DUTY OF CARE

The judge held that a claimant can succeed in a claim against a complementary medicine practitioner either by:[60]

*   calling an expert in the modality in question (this was not done in this case), or
*   proving that the prevailing standard of care and skill in the art in question is deficient in regard to the risks that should have been taken into account.

IMPLICATIONS OF *SHAKOOR V SITU*

The significance of this authority is that:

*   It confirms the approach taken in *Bawden v Marin* that a similar test to that applied to medical doctors will be applied to complementary medicine practitioners; however, it will be based upon the expertise not of a medical practitioner, but rather a reasonably competent member of the complementary medicine modality under consideration.
*   Practitioners are not able to ignore the information and scientific evidence that may be provided by orthodox medicine, which should impact upon the content

of their duty of care to their client. This means, for example, that if an ortho-dox medicine journal describes an adverse event from a complementary medicine procedure (such as chiropractic cervical manipulation) or substance (e.g. adverse reactions to royal jelly), the complementary medicine practitioner may be advised to warn of that risk and take steps to limit the risk of injury.

* It is important in any proceedings brought against a complementary medicine practitioner to obtain expert evidence of what is or is not competent practice for that modality.

The factor that ultimately weighed against the plaintiff in this case was that the adverse reaction was idiosyncratic and not possible to predict.

This authority provides good guidance as to relevant considerations for a negli-gence claim against a complementary medicine practitioner. The application of the varied orthodox medicine standard test—that is, a 'reasonably competent TCM prac-titioner' test—was appropriate on the facts and is consistent with approaches taken in regard to other professions where a profession-specific approach to liability is applied. The inappropriateness of applying the standard of an orthodox medicine practitioner based upon the choice made by the consumer was clear. It is appropriate that the ele-ment of consumer choice in the type of therapy chosen should impact upon the duty of care that is provided. To apply an orthodox medicine standard of care would ignore the different healing philosophy and principles between TCM and orthodox medicine. This approach is given maximum force when the consumer has been provided with adequate information as to the nature of the modality that has been chosen and the implications, risks and advantages of that therapeutic approach.

The application of a modality-specific test permits a balancing of the interests of the practitioner who conforms to standard professional practice and the entitlement of a client to protection from injury. This balancing was in this case provided by the stated necessity for the TCM practitioner to maintain contact with orthodox medicine sources that could impact upon the standard of care required of the TCM practitioner.

BOX 5.6

Practice tip

Practitioners should be aware that the standard of care will change as the general stand-ards of the profession develop over time. What was acceptable practice at the time of graduation may not be acceptable years later. Ensure you keep up to date with issues and innovations in clinical procedures and available technology in your profession.

Applying objective standards to complementary medicine

One issue that will confront a court in assessing the appropriate standard of care is the difficulty of applying objective standards to a modality that relies on a practitioner assessment of the individual circumstances of a client at a particular point in time. Treatment may often be based on the intuitive abilities of a practitioner, which may not always be possible to justify fully on a rational basis.[61] This is in contrast to the more scientific and rational basis used for orthodox medicine procedures.

An expert practitioner of the same modality may have difficulty in asserting, months or years after the initial contact with the client, that the care given was within acceptable practice. Such therapeutic decisions may, in accordance with the parameters of acceptable practice, be made based on the practitioner's perception of subtle energy fluctuations of an individual and intuitive feelings of the practitioner.[62]

The common law model is based on a paternalistic view of orthodox medicine. The doctor as expert 'does something' to or for an essentially passive patient. This type of relationship easily permits the application of tortious liability for negligence when what the doctor did to the patient caused damage. Complementary medicine practitioners may seek to work with clients so that the client has a substantial degree of responsibility for their own healing. The common law test does not easily conform to this type of therapeutic relationship. Despite these difficulties, a court will make an assessment of whether the practitioner has conformed to the standard of care of a reasonably competent practitioner.

The difficulty in applying objective criteria to complementary medicine will be lessened where:

*   the act of the therapist was clearly not what a reasonably competent therapist would do (e.g. where an acupuncturist caused infection by not following proper hygiene practices)[63]
*   there is an obvious connection between the practice involved and the injury suffered (e.g. fractured ribs after chiropractic or osteopathic treatment)[64]
*   there are burns from moxibustion or similar therapy
*   a patient falls from a table because of the practitioner's lack of care in mounting and dismounting
*   there are on-table incidents such as a finger being caught in a treatment table, and
*   the modality is closer to the medical model and the procedures are more standardised (e.g. chiropractic or osteopathy).

The role of medical expert evidence

Is it appropriate for an orthodox medicine practitioner to give evidence in relation to a claim made against a complementary medicine practitioner? This issue arises for a number of reasons:

*   It may be difficult to find an expert complementary medicine practitioner who is prepared to give evidence against a colleague (the conspiracy of silence).
*   The statutory restricted act of 'cervical manipulation', which may only be performed by a chiropractor, osteopath, physiotherapist or medical practitioner, suggests at least a theoretical overlap between the professions.

A US example is the case of *Rosenberg v Rosenberg*.[65] An allegation of negligence was made against a chiropractor because he had failed to recognise tumours shown on an x-ray. The chiropractor noted a 'subluxated vertebra' and recommended manipulation. The claim made was that the failure to diagnose the tumour delayed orthodox treatment. The court accepted medical evidence on the standard of care of chiropractors on the following basis:[66]

The act of negligence must involve the breach of a duty that the medical doctor can evaluate. When the standard of care is within the doctor's field of expertise, and thus is common to both practices, the doctor will be qualified to testify as an expert on that issue.

The use of x-rays in diagnosis by both professions was perceived as the basis of the medical evidence in that case. There is no Australian case specifically on this point. Medical evidence was accepted for the plaintiff in *Bawden v Marin*, which related to the negligence of a chiropractor, although the defendant's expert chiropractor's evidence seems to have been preferred.

There is no indication in *Bawden v Marin* why the court accepted the medical evidence. This is an issue for all complementary medicine practitioners, but especially for those most closely aligned with orthodox medicine, such as chiropractors and osteopaths.

The recent English case of *Shakoor v Situ* (see above) suggests that any claim against a complementary medicine practitioner will require expert evidence from a practitioner of the modality under question. Without such evidence, it may be difficult to demonstrate whether the modality-specific duty of care has been satisfied.

Defences to negligence   .

If all the required elements of negligence are satisfied, the defendant may claim a defence that could avoid or limit liability in some way. The defences may be voluntary assumption of risk, contributory negligence or limitations of actions.

Voluntary assumption of risk

The defence of voluntary assumption of risk (*volenti non fit injuria*) proposes that, as a party has voluntarily undertaken a risk, they absolve the defendant from liability for that risk. If successful, this defence is a complete bar to a negligence claim. The elements of this defence are:

*   The plaintiff had full knowledge of the risk undertaken.
*   The assumption of the risk was voluntary.
*   The risk must be impliedly or expressly waived.

In many cases, it would be difficult to demonstrate all of those elements.[67]

This defence could arise where a client attends a complementary medicine practitioner with a known illness such as heart disease, and accepts treatment. The client may suffer injury as a result of the fact that the practitioner does not (and could not) prescribe drugs normally prescribed by a medical doctor.

A claim for negligence by the client may be met by a defence that the client had voluntarily assumed the risk that only non-medical procedures would be offered by the therapist. The practitioner would argue that they had not been held out as a medical doctor and treated the client within the confines of their profession, thus satisfying their duty of care.

A number of authorities from the United States suggest that this defence is available where a client chooses therapies that do not rely on the orthodox medicine model.

The client cannot then complain if he or she receives the treatment on that basis without reference to orthodox medicine.[68]

The availability of this defence is limited. There are no reported cases in Australia or the United Kingdom that confirm the application of such a defence in medical negligence cases. This was formerly an important defence in general negligence cases, but in recent decades the courts have tended to limit this defence so that it is rarely successful today. Increasingly, the defence of contributory negligence is favoured, as this has the effect of apportioning but not barring recovery. Practitioners should assist the possible application of this defence by advising clients clearly that they should not stop seeking medical advice or taking prescribed drugs, and by clearly indicating the nature of and the limits of the therapy they provide.

The civil liability legislation may assist the use of this defence in a negligence claim. These reforms state that if a defence of voluntary assumption of risk is raised by a defendant, and the risk is obvious (that is, patent or a matter of common knowledge even if the risk has a low probability of occurring and may not be prominent, conspicuous or physically observable), the plaintiff is taken to be aware of the risk, or the type or kind of risk, unless the plaintiff proves on the balance of probabilities that he or she was not aware of it.

Contributory negligence

A client may be deemed to be negligent in his or her own acts, thus reducing the possible claim against a practitioner. Every practitioner can recount instances of negligent, careless acts by clients who have failed to heed instructions and advice, to their detriment. A court generally will be slow to find contributory negligence, and common law principles will require a low standard of behaviour from clients. The civil liability legislation now requires a client to act as a reasonable person would act, based on what that person knew or ought to have known, when considering whether the client has contributed to their injury. This may suggest that the law may now require a somewhat higher standard of behaviour by clients.

An example of contributory negligence in the medical sphere was where a client obtained further drugs beyond the initial prescription, and suffered loss of sight as a result.[69] In this case, the patient was held to be two-thirds to blame. In another case, a diabetic client failed to follow a prescribed diet, allowing contributory negligence to be a defence.[70]

This defence is often not available in the medical context on the basis of the power disparity between doctor and patient. The doctor is perceived as 'all knowing' and the patient as relying on the instructions and skill of the doctor. This is not the type of therapeutic relationship that complementary medicine practitioners normally seek to engender. This might support a broader application of contributory negligence in that context.

Practitioners should make sure that clients understand clinical instructions, and should properly monitor for compliance. For remedial exercises, a practitioner should remember that a client may not be accustomed to complex instructions.[71] A patient could undertake the wrong exercises or perform them in a way that causes injury. This suggests that a client should be given proper instruction in writing and asked to perform the exercises before leaving the clinic, with a follow-up on the next visit to ensure proper understanding and compliance.

The civil liability legislation in New South Wales (s 5S), Victoria (s 63) and Queensland (s 24) provides that contributory negligence may be a complete defence, while in the other jurisdictions contributory negligence can only reduce the amount of damages recoverable in any claim.

Limitation period

There is a specified period of time within which a negligence action must be commenced, otherwise the action is 'statute barred'. This period may be extended in the case of disability such as mental illness, and will not commence until a party reaches eighteen years of age. The period will run from the damage being suffered, which will often be the date of the negligent act but may be later. For example, the damage done from a negligent manipulation may manifest years later.

Apologies and statements of regret

When an adverse or unexpected result of treatment occurs, it may be considered appropriate to provide an apology or statement of regret to the client. A client may be less likely to lodge a complaint or to commence legal action if they consider a practitioner has been genuine in their attempts to perform their professional tasks competently. An expression of regret or apology may be beneficial in dealing with a difficult situation. This action may, however, have legal implications if it is perceived as an admission of liability. For this reason, reference to the professional indemnity insurer or to legal advice may be advisable before any such statements are made. The civil liability legislation now provides some protection for such statements in some circumstances, although care is still required.

In New South Wales, under sections 68 and 69 of the *Civil Liability Act 2002*, an apology means an expression of sympathy or regret or of a general sense of benevolence or compassion in connection with any matter, whether or not the apology admits or implies an admission of fault in connection with the matter. Thus in New South Wales an apology is not considered an admission of guilt and is not admissible in any claim. The ACT provides similarly.

In Queensland, under sections 68–72 of the *Civil Liability Act 2003*, an expression of regret made by an individual in relation to an incident alleged to give rise to an action for damages means any oral or written statement expressing regret for the incident to the extent that it does not contain an admission of liability on the part of the individual or someone else. An expression of regret as defined is not admissible evidence.

In Victoria, under sections 14I–14L of the *Wrongs Act 1958*, an apology means an expression of sorrow, regret or sympathy, but does not include a clear acknowledgement of fault. Tasmania, the Northern Territory and Western Australia provide similarly. An apology as defined is not admissible evidence.

Accordingly, in Queensland, Victoria, Western Australia, Tasmania and the Northern Territory, an apology that contains an admission of guilt may be admissible in any claim made against that person. This suggests that great care should be taken to ensure any expression of regret does not include an acknowledgement of guilt.

BOX 5.7

Practice tip: The risky client

Practitioners need to identify clients who might trigger a professional liability claim. Campbell categorises clients who require special care as follows:[72]

- The complainer. A client who is vociferous in complaints against doctors, hospitals and other professionals may have a proper basis for his or her complaints. It could also be a pattern of complaints about treatment, which will rarely meet their expectations. These clients may be a source of an unjustified claim for negligence or professional misconduct, and should be dealt with carefully.
- The touter. This client may exclaim the virtues of the practitioner, indicating that he has heard that the practitioner can help when no one else could. This may be a client who has unrealistic expectations that inevitably will be deflated.
- The fanatic. This client may be an adherent to the latest fads, diets and philosophies, who in switching from fad to fad may quickly consider you to be out of fashion.
- The responsibility shifter. This is a client who considers that it is your job to heal them, and their role to be healed. This client may not be open to advice on lifestyle issues as an important part of the healing process, and may not understand that the practitioner is primarily helping the body to heal itself. This patient may be less likely to follow instructions and more likely to become dissatisfied if quick progress is not demonstrated.
- The dishonest client. The client who asks openly about defrauding, or insinuates that he or she would like to defraud a medical benefits fund or their employer in regard to their condition, may also be dishonest in their dealings with you.
- Clients with a susceptibility to injury. An example might be a client with osteoporosis or arthritis. If necessary, x-ray evidence may be required to rule out treatments or manipulations that may be dangerous. Chiropractors and osteopaths need care in giving manipulations without proper investigation for hidden fractures or injuries that could be exacerbated. Special susceptibility to herbs or oils should be ascertained prior to treatment, and a record of this made on the patient's file. A practitioner can choose not to treat a client who has a susceptibility that makes them too great a risk to treat.

Who is liable?

If treatment by a complementary medicine practitioner causes injury, a number of persons may be liable. These could include:

- the manufacturer of faulty equipment or substances that caused the injury, such as faulty acupuncture needles or an adulterated herbal mixture
- the treating healthcare professional, and
- an employer of the employee healthcare professional responsible for the injury.

A plaintiff may choose to sue all or some of these persons. The choice of which party should be proceeded against may depend on which potential defendant has assets sufficient to satisfy any claim. This may be determined by whether the defendant has professional indemnity insurance to satisfy any claim.

Each defendant is potentially liable for the whole of the damages awarded in a case. If one party satisfies the judgement, there may be a claim for a contribution from other defendants.[73]

Providing services on behalf of a third party

A practitioner may be engaged to provide services to a person on behalf of a third party, who is likely to be paying for such services. This may occur where:

- treatment is provided pursuant to workers compensation legislation
- there is an examination for an insurance company (e.g. to confirm the extent of injury or prognosis), and
- a health clearance is sought by an employer in relation to a prospective employee.

This type of task will usually be performed by medical doctors, but may be part of the role of a chiropractor or osteopath and, in some states, massage therapists for workers' compensation.

What is the duty of care in these circumstances?

- *Third-party client.* The practitioner's duty is to provide professional services at the standard of a reasonably competent practitioner. The practitioner may be liable in negligence or in contract for any damages suffered by the third-party client for errors in the assessment of the person examined or for injury caused by the examination. An employer may rely on a health report before employing a person who is not fit for service.
- *Person examined.* The case law on this point is limited. A practitioner may be liable for injury caused by a negligent examination or by errors in diagnosis. If the practitioner diagnoses a serious complaint, the practitioner may be obliged to advise the person examined of the diagnosis and the need to seek treatment. Liability to the person examined may also arise for the non-diagnosis or wrong diagnosis of a condition that the practitioner should have found using the tests requested.[74] It may be doubted whether the duty of care would extend beyond dealing with tests expressly requested by the third-party client.

Abandonment

In the United States, medical doctors and chiropractors have been found liable for abandonment of clients, causing injury. Abandonment is not a distinct head of liability in Australia, but liability could arise based on a breach of the general duty of care. It is good professional practice to ensure that a client is not left without reasonable access to necessary treatment.

The US authorities indicate that liability can arise for abandonment where a plaintiff can show that:[75]

- the practitioner owed a duty to the plaintiff
- the practitioner's withdrawal of services was unilateral
- the patient was in need of continued treatment

- the client sustained injury as a result of the non-availability of treatment, and
- the practitioner's abandonment caused the injury.

Possible liability for abandonment could occur when:

- withdrawing professional services on the basis that the patient is uncooperative or abusive
- the practitioner retires
- the practitioner is on vacation or absent for other reasons, or
- the practitioner changes his or her place of business.

A practitioner is entitled to terminate a therapeutic relationship if there is a personality conflict, because the patient cannot be assisted by the treatment provided, if the required treatment is beyond the practitioner's scope of practice or for other reasons. This is especially relevant for medical doctors where a seriously ill patient may be unable to secure medical services before their condition worsens. This situation would apply rarely for complementary medicine practitioners.

Note that under the AHPRA Code of Conduct clause 4.11 suggests that when closing or relocating a practice advance notice should be given to patients. In addition, arrangements should be made for continuing care of current patients and the transfer of health records in accordance with privacy obligations.

BOX 5.8

Practice tip: Withdrawal of services

If a practitioner is contemplating withdrawal of professional services, they should give reasonable notice to the client so that they are able to engage another practitioner. What is reasonable notice would depend on circumstances such as the state of health of the client and the availability of other practitioners.

When a practice is relocated any distance or retirement is contemplated, it would be advisable to give notice to each client individually and to indicate that you could refer them to other practitioners in the locality. If selling a practice to another practitioner, an introduction to the new owner is advisable and may be a contractual obligation of the sale of business contract.

If the client chooses to terminate services (this may be in acrimonious circumstances), to avoid a claim of abandonment or breach of duty it would be advisable to note that the termination of services was the client's decision. A confirmatory letter indicating whether further treatment is needed and suggesting other possible practitioners would provide the best protection for a cautious practitioner.

Referral to medical practitioner or other practitioner

A client is entitled to choose the health practitioner or modality they want and can freely choose complementary medicine over orthodox medicine, and a complementary medicine practitioner is entitled to provide that treatment subject to legal and ethical restraints and their qualifications and training. A client should be provided with information to understand the nature of treatment being offered and should, in appropriate cases, be referred for medical treatment or other forms of treatment. The Codes of Conduct for Unregistered Health Practitioners prohibit a holding out of the capacity to treat or cure cancer but permit a claim about their ability or willingness to treat or alleviate the symptoms of those illnesses if that claim can be substantiated. The Code also requires a client not to be discouraged from continuing medical treatment. Refer to these Codes above pages 82–92.

Potential civil and criminal liability for failure to refer

A person will usually consult a complementary medicine practitioner to obtain services of a different nature from those offered by a medical practitioner. If a client suffers damage that would not have occurred if the client had been appropriately referred to a medical practitioner, the client may argue that the practitioner has liability in negligence for that injury for a breach of a duty of care to refer to a medical practitioner when that was within the duty of care of that practitioner and the referral could be demonstrated to avoid any injury to the client. A medical practitioner may be liable in negligence if he or she fails to refer to a specialist when an issue arises that the practitioner is not able to diagnose or treat and the failure to refer is found to have caused damage to the patient.[76] Although there is no clear judicial authority on this point, the court will be likely to respect the therapeutic choices made by a client but may consider that a duty to refer to another health practitioner may arise for a complementary medicine practitioner in some circumstances. Each circumstance is different and this may vary depending on the level of training and qualification of the practitioner and the nature of the malady considered; however, care needs to be exercised.

A defence to this claim could be that the client voluntarily undertook non-medical treatment and understood the type of therapy that was being undertaken. This was a factor in the English case of *Shakoor v Situ*, where a judge determined not to apply the standard of care of an orthodox medicine practitioner for a claim made against a Chinese medicine practitioner as the client had chosen to use Chinese medicine and not orthodox medicine (for more detail, refer to pages 108–113 above).

The practitioner is placed in a stronger ethical and legal position if he or she does not advise against the patient seeking medical advice and the client clearly understands the nature of the service provided, including its risks and level of efficacy. If the circumstances are reviewed, a court would be likely to consider issues such as the seriousness of the illness under consideration, whether there was clarity about the nature of the illness or injury being treated, whether the complementary medicine practitioner was acting as the primary health practitioner, whether there was a medical diagnosis available (which may or may not be correct), the level of training of the practitioner and whether there was a patent or possible indication of some underlying pathology beyond the scope of practice of the practitioner. A court may take into account the vulnerable position of a client and the possibility of undue influence by the practitioner.

To avoid potential liability and to protect the interests of the client, a practitioner should refer to a medical doctor or other appropriate practitioner a client with a malady that initially or subsequently patently requires medical or some other form of treatment or does not respond to the practitioner's modality, which may suggest some underlying pathology beyond the scope of practice or training of the practitioner. Alternatively, the practitioner may seek to treat the client in a complementary manner while the client obtains advice from an orthodox medical or some other appropriate practitioner. An obvious example where a referral is required is a client with a fractured bone or suspected fractured bone, or a client with a potentially serious illness such as cancer, diabetes, heart disease or serious infection, or a client with a condition that requires further investigation or testing. A court may consider that those types of illnesses or injuries require medical attention, though in appropriate cases treatment of the symptoms of serious illness may be appropriate if it is within the scope of practice, training and qualifications of the practitioner. The identification of these diseases and states may be relatively simple for practitioners who have the required training in diagnosis and analysis of disease states, but more difficult for others. The lack of access to sophisticated diagnostic equipment suggests that complementary practitioners have a duty of care to be aware of the possibility of an underlying and undiagnosed injury or disease that may impact on the nature of suitable treatment and the need to refer to a medical doctor or other appropriate health practitioner.

A practitioner might be entitled to continue treatment while medical advice is obtained, if the treatment will not aggravate the condition. If the practitioner decides to treat and the client's condition worsens or there is no improvement, the practitioner should consider whether a referral to a medical doctor should then be made. This referral should be made early rather than late. A practitioner would be in a precarious position in relation to civil liability for negligence if, on the advice of a complementary medicine practitioner, a client failed to seek medical assistance and the passage of time meant that the chance of successful medical treatment was lost. Although the case law on liability for loss of a chance to receive treatment suggests courts are slow to find liability for 'loss of chance', if it can be established that a failure to refer has caused injury, this may raise potential liability in negligence.[77]

There have been a number of recent cases involving complementary medicine practitioners in Australia where criminal convictions have resulted from a failure to refer a client for medical care at all, or when the referral was delayed so as to result in a negative outcome for the client.

In Australia, an eighteen-day-old baby had a serious heart defect, which was apparently curable with a surgical procedure that had a high success rate. A naturopath advised the parents that, after giving homoeopathic and herbal treatment, the baby was cured of the complaint. On the basis of the advice of the naturopath, the parents chose not to proceed with surgery. The baby died shortly afterwards. The practitioner was convicted of manslaughter.[78]

A Melbourne naturopath advised the parents of a boy to stop chemotherapy that had a 60 per cent chance of success. The boy died six months later, three days after the parents had requested that chemotherapy be restarted.[79]

In New South Wales, a father and mother of a child were convicted of manslaughter after the death of their infant child who had suffered from complications associated with serious eczema. The parents (the father was a homoeopath) relied on homoeopathy with limited use of orthodox medicine. Although there was adequate access to orthodox medicine to deal with this condition, and the parents received advice that orthodox medicine was required for treatment, this medical warning was not heeded. The child eventually died from infection and malnutrition, although it was likely that this result would have been avoided by appropriate orthodox medicine intervention.[80]

In the US case of *Ison v McFall*,[81] a workman experienced weakness and numbness in his back after chiropractic manipulations. Despite these symptoms, the chiropractor continued treatment. The client eventually lost the use of his legs and bodily function as a result of an undiagnosed tumour. The chiropractor in that instance was deemed liable for negligence because he didn't refer the patient for medical treatment.

Some US authorities suggest that a chiropractor should identify conditions that are not amenable to chiropractic and require medical treatment. The practitioner should refrain from further treatment if it will aggravate or not improve the client's condition and refer to a medical doctor or at least indicate that chiropractic cannot assist the client.[82] This general approach would be suitable for other complementary medicine practitioners.

Bearing in mind the less extensive training in diagnosis for many complementary medicine practitioners, it is hoped that a court would be more forgiving of a failure to identify a difficult-to-diagnose medical problem. The court would most likely expect a practitioner to refer to a doctor where a client failed to respond or continued to worsen while under the practitioner's care. This necessity should be obvious in many cases, even to those modalities not trained in diagnosis of disease states.

BOX 5.9

Practice tip

What should a practitioner do in this fact scenario?

A client attends your acupuncture clinic. She tells you she has been diagnosed with inoperable liver cancer. Her medical prognosis is likely death within six months. She asks you to treat her as she has no other medical options. A practitioner should not suggest he or she have an ability to cure cancer, especially in New South Wales, Victoria, Queensland and South Australia where the Code of Conduct for Unregistered Health Practitioners prohibits it.

Any treatment of symptoms of terminal illnesses must be able to be substantiated. The treatment of a serious illness such as cancer is more likely to cause concern for regulators and for the client's friends and relatives regarding the appropriateness of the treatment. If treating a person in this circumstance, consider the following procedures:

- Advise the client that any treatment is not for treating the cancer but for the improvement in the client's general health, if that statement is justified based upon your clinical training.
- Require the client to keep in contact with their medical doctor.
- Never discourage a client from seeking medical advice or continuing medical treatment.
- Never claim the ability to cure or treat cancer.
- A letter to the client confirming the above would be advisable.
- Have evidence that the claim to treat in this manner can be substantiated.

Providing information to clients

A client will be more cooperative and likely to conform to clinical aims if they are properly advised of what to expect in the healing process. Practitioners need to inform clients to the full extent possible of any risks of treatment. Without proper warnings of risk, an unexpected outcome may provide the basis for a claim for negligence against the practitioner even if competent treatment is given. Open, honest and thorough communication with your client is the key. A client is entitled to make decisions reflecting the ethical principle of autonomy.

Warnings of risk

If a practitioner fails to give a client sufficient warning of potential risks of treatment, the practitioner may be deemed negligent by allowing a person to undertake a procedure without the opportunity to give proper consent to that treatment. This has been described as a 'rigorous legal obligation' and is based on 'the paramount consideration that a person is entitled to make his own decisions about his life'.[83]

This issue is particularly important in medical practice, which may involve complex surgery and medicinal regimes carrying potentially lethal outcomes and complications. The nature of complementary medicine suggests that it will be rare for a client to be faced with potentially drastic outcomes of therapy. However, the obligation to warn of risks of treatment should still be observed, as it also applies to less dramatic treatment risks.

Rogers v Whitaker

This issue was highlighted by the High Court decision in *Rogers v Whitaker*.[84] In this case, Mrs Whitaker sought the advice of Mr Rogers, an ophthalmic surgeon. Mrs Whitaker was blind in her right eye as the result of a childhood accident. She approached the doctor about an operation to improve the appearance and sight function of that eye. Before the operation, Mrs Whitaker was very concerned that the doctor might by error operate on her good eye and about the possible result of the operation. After the operation, the bad eye did not improve but the left eye developed sympathetic ophthalmia, causing almost total blindness. This complication had a risk factor of only one in 14,000 procedures. The surgeon had not warned Mrs Whitaker of this complication on the basis that it was a very remote possibility. Importantly, expert evidence presented to the court supported the view that the approach was in accordance with accepted medical procedures.

The High Court indicated that the court, not the profession, determined what advice and information as to risks should be provided to a client. The court stated:[85]

> while evidence of acceptable medical practice is a useful guide for the courts, it is for the courts to adjudicate on what is the appropriate standard of care after giving weight to the paramount consideration that a person is entitled to make his own decisions about his life.

On these facts, despite the fact that medical opinion favoured not revealing the possible complication, the doctor was found negligent. The appropriate test to apply for a doctor was:[86]

a doctor has a duty to warn a patient of a material risk inherent in the proposed treatment; a risk is material if, in the circumstances of the particular case, a reasonable person in the patient's position, if warned of the risk would be likely to attach significance to it or if the medical practitioner is or should reasonably be aware that the particular patient, if warned of the risk, would be likely to attach significance to it.

The important factors in this case were that the patient was clearly very concerned about possible complications and the potential for a drastic outcome if there was any negative impact on the good eye. For the court, this suggested that, despite medical opinion to the contrary, the doctor was negligent to fail to warn of this risk of the treatment.

The court concluded that Mrs Whitaker would not have proceeded with the treatment if she had been alerted to this possible complication. This requires the court to look at what that patient would have done if they had received the proper warning, despite the obvious risk that a recollection of events will often be coloured by the damage that the patient later suffers.

Chappel v Hart

The obligation to warn of risks was broadened in the High Court case of *Chappel v Hart*.[87] Here, the High Court concluded that a doctor was negligent in failing to warn of a rare complication (damaged vocal cords) of oesophagus surgery.

Despite evidence confirming that the doctor did not perform the surgery negligently, the doctor was deemed negligent for a failure to warn of this complication. The doctor argued that he was not liable, as the damage could have happened despite his lack of warning as the patient would have required the surgery eventually. As it was a random event, the damage to the vocal cord may still have happened. The High Court by majority concluded that the patient would not have had the surgery by the defendant doctor if warned about the risk of this complication. Important to this finding was the fact that, as a relatively inexperienced surgeon, there was a greater chance of this complication than with the most experienced surgeons. If properly warned, the patient might have used a more experienced doctor, which would have reduced the possibility of such a complication. It was the loss of the chance to use the more experienced surgeon that was the basis of the liability. These authorities suggest a very broad obligation on medical doctors to warn of risks.

Impact of civil liability legislation on duty to warn of risks

The civil liability legislation in most states provides that the duty of care of a professional discussed above does not impact on the duty to advise of risks of treatment. This means that a complementary medicine practitioner, if deemed a 'professional' under these provisions, cannot avoid liability by stating that he or she was relying on standard professional practice when not providing adequate warning of the risks of treatment.

Accordingly, the common law principles discussed above will be at least generally relevant in many situations. Some jurisdictions have specific provisions in relation to advising of risks of treatment. For example, in Victoria under section 50 of the *Wrongs Act 1958*, a duty to warn is satisfied if the defendant takes reasonable care in giving that warning or other information.

BOX 5.10

Practice tip: Complementary medicine—warnings of risk

The above authorities suggest a broad obligation on complementary medicine practitioners to inform clients of risks of treatment. The possible risks of treatment might be symptoms such as:[88]

- fainting
- headaches
- tiredness
- possible adverse reactions
- reactions to pharmaceuticals
- bruising
- scarring
- menstrual disturbance
- nausea/vomiting, or
- conditions becoming worse before improvement.

Although a client may be prepared to accept these often mild reactions as a price for the treatment, a practitioner should warn a client of possible outcomes of treatment. The client could argue that, if told of the possible side-effects, they would not have undertaken the offered treatment. When a medical doctor is dealing with a serious illness such as heart disease or cancer, it may be difficult for a plaintiff to demonstrate that if they were given the appropriate warnings they would not have undertaken the treatment. Where a medical patient is considering a risky but potentially life-saving operation, a court may conclude that, despite inadequate warnings, the patient would still have decided to continue with the procedure. In this case, the practitioner would not be liable for negligence in failing to inform of the risk that eventuated.[89]

The same could not be said about a less serious ailment or chronic condition that may be presented to a complementary medicine practitioner. A client might wish to seek other options without the attendant risk. It may be more difficult to argue that the client would have proceeded anyway, even if the risks were fully described.[90]

This suggests that a complementary medicine practitioner should provide clients with enough information to allow them to make a decision about whether or not to proceed with treatment. Quite apart from the issue of potential legal liability, good professional practice dictates full disclosure to clients of treatments contemplated and the communication of intended results and possible outcomes.

Defence to wrongful non-disclosure

A practitioner may argue that the risk of a negative outcome is so low that it is not necessary to mention it to a client. The determination that a risk did not require a warning would depend on the current state of scientific knowledge and all the relevant circumstances of the case. In *Rogers v Whitaker*, the risk of complication that occurred (blindness in the eye that was not operated on) was calculated as one in 14,000 but in the circumstances the High Court considered it a risk that should have been revealed. In different contexts, the duty to warn of risks will vary depending on the nature of the risk, the client under consideration and the general circumstances.

Advising of alternative therapies

If a client attends a practitioner with a condition that may respond to medical treatment, is the practitioner required to indicate the possibility of medical alternatives?

A medical doctor may be liable for adverse results if he or she fails to indicate other treatment options such as pain relief, traction or rest when suggesting treatments such as surgery. If given an option, the client may choose a less radical procedure without the attendant risks.

To require complementary medicine practitioners to advise of medical treatment options would be unreasonable, as this is not within their professional purview. The broad obligation for medical doctors to discuss treatment options is because they are primary health practitioners entitled to provide virtually any therapy for the alleviation of ailments and diseases. In their professional practice, complementary medicine practitioners are excluded from restricted acts by statute, or by limits in training, experience and knowledge. Within their area of practice, complementary medicine practitioners should ensure that options for treatment and the risks of that treatment are discussed with a client so that the client can select the one they prefer.

Practitioners should also understand their limitations. If a client presents with a condition such as diabetes or cancer that is best dealt with by a medical practitioner, the practitioner should advise the client to seek medical assistance. If, after appropriate advice, the client chooses not to seek medical treatment, this should be noted on the client's file. The client should also be advised of any limitations of the treatment provided. A letter confirming this advice is the best evidence that the client has been so informed. It is also important for a practitioner to be quick to refer a client whose condition is not improving or is worsening, or where the practitioner does not understand the presentation of the disease or its implications. Refer to the Ethical Protocol for Complementary Medicine Practitioners at pages 27–28.

The Osteopathy Board of Australia Informed Consent: Guidelines for Osteopaths, April 2013, provided a good overview of the information that should be provided to clients to provide adequate informed consent:

In order to provide informed consent a patient has a right to sufficient information for his/her understanding of:[91]

1 the diagnosis and likely outcome (prognosis) of the condition
2 an explanation of the recommended treatment
3 the risks of the procedure and common side effects
4 possible complications
5 specific details of the treatment
6 any other options for treatment and their probability of success
7 cost of treatment
8 option to defer treatment, and
9 right to withdraw consent to treatment at any time.

In addition, it is advisable to discuss the likely pain or suffering involved (if any, such as soreness) at the time of obtaining the consent. It is important to take measures to ensure the client is able to understand the information provided to them by using easily understood language; repeating information if required; permitting questions;

providing time to make decisions; and, if necessary, providing translation services or family members or carers to assist in understanding.

Therapeutic privilege

The concept of therapeutic privilege[92] may permit a doctor to withhold information from a patient because that information would be to the detriment of the patient. This might occur where, because of the patient's personality or level of understanding and the nature of treatment, the information would cause such distress as to harm the patient.[93] This is a privilege that applies only rarely in medical practice. There is no authority to suggest that this privilege would apply to complementary medicine, and the nature of complementary medicine suggests that it is difficult to justify this privilege being claimed.[94]

Consent to treatment

It is fundamental to a just and ethical society that people are autonomous and able to control their bodies and what others are permitted to do to their bodies. It is for the client, not the practitioner, to determine whether and when any procedure or treatment should occur. Consent to treatment (which may be express or implied) should be voluntarily and freely given, based on competent and truthful advice pitched at the appropriate level of comprehension for that client so that a client can understand the specific nature of the act to which they are consenting. A client who provides consent to treatment after proper advice will be more cooperative, trusting and likely to follow instructions.[95] Consent can only be obtained from a person who is competent to give consent.

Trespass to the person

The law protects the ability of a person to choose by whom and how they are touched. If a practitioner touches a client without their consent, the practitioner may be liable for trespass to the person and negligence.

Trespass to the person incorporates civil assault and battery. Civil assault is apprehension of physical harm, while battery is the application of physical force to a person. Not obtaining proper consent to treatment may also create liability in negligence or professional misconduct, and in serious cases even criminal assault.

The need for consent to touch a client is fundamental for a complementary medicine practitioner as bodily contact is necessary for examinations, the insertion of an acupuncture needle, massage or spinal manipulations. Consent turns a potential battery into a legally permissible touching.[96]

Liability for battery will be avoided if the client consents to the touching after the practitioner gives the client basic information on the general nature of the touching. This issue will arise most clearly when the touching goes beyond that contemplated by the consenting party. This might occur where the touching is deemed to be of a sexual nature, or where there was consent for one type of procedure such as a chiropractic manipulation when in fact an entirely different procedure is applied, such as insertion of an acupuncture needle. Practitioners should never proceed with treatment in the absence of clear consent.

How can consent be given?

Consent can be given either expressly or impliedly.

Express consent

- *Written.* A practitioner may obtain express written consent to a procedure from a client. A chiropractor might explain in writing the nature of the manipulations intended and the physical impact of those manipulations, such as the sounds made and any possible side-effects. The client could then consent in writing to those procedures. Refer to the discussion on pages 128–129 on the role of written consent forms.
- *Verbal express consent.* After an explanation is given of the intended treatment, a client may verbally consent to the procedure. For example, an acupuncturist might indicate that a number of needles would be sited in particular parts of the body, and describe the physical sensations that would be felt and the impact of the procedure. The patient could then consent verbally to this procedure. This form of consent will commonly be relied upon by practitioners.
- *Implied consent.* After a description is made of the procedures intended, if a client lies on a treatment couch, removes their clothes in preparation for a massage or proffers their arm or body for the insertion of an acupuncture needle, this normally will indicate implied consent. Consent will often be obtained by this method.

This consent could be rebutted if it were shown that the implied consent was for some other procedure (for example, if the client was expecting a chiropractic manipulation but the touching involved the use of moxibustion therapy). Practitioners should ensure that any consent granted by the client is voluntary, not coerced or promoted by fraudulent means, and relates to the procedures actually performed on the client.

Consent in a continuing therapeutic relationship

In the context of a continuing therapeutic relationship, is a separate consent required on each visit or when each new technique is applied?

Whether proper consent has been obtained will be based on a common-sense assessment of all the circumstances. Most of the authorities dealing with a lack of consent relate to instances where a medical doctor performs, often in the context of an operation, a different procedure to that contemplated by the client. These are clear cases.

More difficult cases arise where, for example, a client has been attending a practitioner for some time and undergoing similar procedures.

- *Consent where course of treatment is specified.* If a patient has consented to a course of treatment, such as a specified number of acupuncture treatments over a number of weeks, it would be easy to imply consent for the procedures at each visit based simply on the client's arrival for the treatment. Despite this probable protection, a practitioner should remind the client of what is contemplated at the beginning of each visit.
- *Consent where a new type of therapy is introduced.* If a new type of therapy or procedure is contemplated (e.g. instead of using needles, the practitioner intends to use moxibustion), a separate consent should be obtained for the procedure even

if it had been discussed on a previous visit. The consent should involve discussion of the nature of the procedure and any relevant risks of that procedure.

- *Consent where a succession of techniques is employed.* During the consultation, a chiropractor may use hand manipulation of the neck, manipulation of the lumbar region, manipulations using the table and instruments, therapeutic massage and then kinesiology. Should a series of explanations of the procedure and consent be obtained at each stage? This could involve a time-consuming and somewhat impractical requirement for practitioners.

Consent probably should be obtained at each stage, subject to a common-sense appraisal of the client based on considerations such as:

- whether the client has previously received this type of treatment
- previous indications by the client of the type of treatment they do or do not want (e.g. they may have indicated that needle insertion should not occur), and
- the dangers and risks of treatment and the explanations previously given to the client.

If what is contemplated has never been explained, a separate consent should be obtained for each procedure. The client should be given the opportunity to indicate after explanation (whether orally, in writing or implicitly) that they consent to the contemplated procedure. The client should not be ambushed and suddenly find themselves subject to a form of treatment not contemplated.

Stone and Matthews[97] express the view that:

> Consent should not be regarded by practitioners as a one-off 'tick in the box', which gives them carte blanche to treat as they see fit. Rather, consent should be viewed as part of an ongoing, dynamic process, which recognizes the patient's ongoing cooperation and willingness to participate in treatment.

Written consent forms

A practitioner may request a client to sign a written consent form containing an explanation of a procedure and details of the risk involved. Other forms may refer to the general nature of treatment to be given. Such documents should be couched in clear and non-technical language to maximise the level of understanding of the person reading or signing the document.

The benefit of completing such a form is that it provides some evidence that an explanation or information has been given to the client. If properly used, it may have the effect of focusing the minds of practitioner and client on the procedures being contemplated. A practitioner may be in a better legal position with such a form than without it. However, the level of protection provided by such forms should not be over-estimated for the following reasons:

- *The court may read against the practitioner.* A court will tend to read these forms against the party who attempts to rely on them. If there is any ambiguity in the way they can be interpreted, a court may interpret them favourably for a client. If this document is interpreted as a 'consumer contract' as defined by the Australian

Consumer Law discussed at pages 158–159, this contract may not be enforceable if the practitioner has not provided reasonable opportunity to negotiate the terms of that contract.

- *Information has not actually been imparted.* The form may be accepted as indicating that the form was signed but not whether any particular information was actually imparted. A client may later suggest that they did not understand the explanation or the form, that they lacked sufficient proficiency in English, or that little time was given for thought or consideration. The best practice would be to personally ask the client to consider the terms of the document and provide them with an oral overview of its terms; provide time for the client to consider the document, to ask questions and to raise any terms or issues they don't understand before placing their signature on the document denoting that they have read and understood the terms of the document. If these steps have been followed in the presence of the client, a practitioner may indicate by a signature that these steps have been followed. It should be remembered that some persons may have difficulty with reading, in comprehension or understanding the English language that they do not want to reveal to a practitioner, so being aware of that possibility is important. Translation services, assistance from a family member or resort to oral information may assist with this process.

- *The signature has been witnessed.* The fact the signature on the form is witnessed is only proof that the form was signed in the presence of the witness and does not by itself add significance to the document. The witness may be able to provide some evidence of what occurred at that time, and this could assist a practitioner.

Who can consent?

Consent to treatment can only be given by a person who is competent to consent. Every adult is presumed competent unless there is evidence or knowledge to the contrary. 'A competent adult is one who is capable of understanding the nature, consequence and risks of a proposed procedure and the consequences of refusing treatment.'[98] A mentally competent person over the age of eighteen years is able to consent to treatment. Persons who have not yet attained the age of eighteen years are minors[99] and are deemed to be under a disability, though children over the age of sixteen years of age are normally considered capable of giving valid consent to treatment.[100]

Adults who are not competent

If an adult is not able to understand the nature of treatment being offered because of mental illness, temporary decision-making incapacity or impairment caused by drugs, it is not possible to obtain consent to treatment from that person. If the incapacity is temporary, a practitioner should delay obtaining consent until capacity is restored or seek consent from a legally appointed guardian or a validly appointed medical agent under an enduring power of attorney. Although complementary medicine is unlikely to be emergency treatment or life-saving, some care is required to ensure that you are obtaining consent from a person who is entitled to give that consent. This is a complex area of law that varies from jurisdiction to jurisdiction, and in terms of specific court orders and powers of attorney. If there is any doubt, specific legal advice may be required or treatment should not be provided.

Parental consent

Failure to obtain valid consent may make a practitioner liable to the possible civil and criminal sanctions relevant to treatment without consent. If a minor cannot give valid consent to treatment, it must be obtained from a parent, guardian or other appropriate person who has the power to consent to procedures that are in the best interests of a child.

Section 61C of the *Family Law Act 1975* (Cth) grants each parent (whether married or not) parental responsibility for a child up to the age of eighteen years to the extent to which it is not displaced by a parenting order made by the Family Court of Australia. Normally these parental powers are vested in both parents jointly, but where there is no indication of a conflict between the parents, a practitioner can usually act on the consent of one parent.[101]

The responsibility given to the parent of a child formally ends at eighteen years, but this is a dwindling right that gradually disappears as the child becomes older. A child of sixteen years is usually deemed capable of providing a valid consent to treatment.

Is a practitioner able to accept consent for treatment from a client who has not attained the age of sixteen years? Legislation in New South Wales[102] permits minors over the age of fourteen years to consent to medical or dental treatment. This provision does not refer to complementary medicine, but provides some indication of the minimum appropriate age for valid consent.

Common law on consent by minors

As no statute provides clear guidance, it is necessary to refer to the common law. The High Court of Australia in *Secretary, Department of Health and Community Services v JWB and SMB* (*Marion*'s case)[103] followed an English decision of *Gillick v West Norfolk and Wisbech Area Health Authority.*[104] The *Gillick* case confirmed that:[105]

> the parental right to determine whether or not their minor child below 16 years will have medical treatment terminates when the child achieves a sufficient understanding and intelligence to enable him or her to understand fully what is proposed.

The *Gillick* test suggests that if a minor can fully understand the nature of the contemplated treatment, then he or she is competent to consent.[106] This test is a difficult one to apply in practice. The practitioner must assess the level of maturity and understanding of a client to determine whether they can validly consent to treatment. Important criteria are matters such as:

*   cognitive development
*   whether the child is still living with and under the supervision of parents, and
*   the nature of the treatment being contemplated.

As complementary medicine is unlikely to involve major risks of complications or have a lasting impact on the client's life, this might suggest that a more robust approach to this issue is justified. The Western Australia Law Reform Commission, however, concluded that the same considerations applied to complementary medicine as were appropriate in medical or allied medical cases.[107] Stone and Matthews argue similarly that a court, which is normally conservative in approach, may tend to favour medical treatment, thus increasing the onus of proof to show a valid consent by a minor for complementary medicine treatment.[108] Accordingly, the cautious approach for a practitioner is to require the consent of parents for treatment in all children up to the age of sixteen years.

Disagreement between parents and child

If a child is competent to give consent, the parent or guardian cannot countermand this. If the parents have consented to treatment but the child refuses, it would seem to follow that a child with sufficient maturity to consent can resist the procedure. There is some doubt about this position where life-saving medical procedures are required and the minor does not consent. A complementary medicine practitioner will rarely provide acute care in such a situation, but a practitioner may in this situation be advised to await a court order allowing the treatment that the child has refused to undertake.

Special care needs to be taken when a child under sixteen years gives consent to treatment for a condition that arguably might require medical intervention. A court may take a tougher line on the obligation to obtain consent from the parent in that circumstance.[109]

Liability in contract

In many instances where an injury is alleged to have occurred in regard to medical treatment, there may in addition be liability in contract.[110] A client may commence the action in tort and contract, though only one set of damages would be recoverable if liability were proven. Liability in contract may occur in two circumstances: express contract and implied contract.

Express contract

An express contract, either written or oral, may involve an undertaking for specific services and/or a promise of a particular result. If the services are not provided or the result contracted for is not obtained, there may be liability in contract for damages.

If the promised result does not eventuate, the practitioner may be liable for a refund of professional fees paid and possibly other damages. This obligation will arise even if the services have been provided without negligence, as the basis of liability is the contract to provide a specific result. It is clearly important not to guarantee a result or 'cure' unless the practitioner is prepared for possible liability in contract for damages if the contract is not satisfied.[111]

Some practitioners may ask clients to sign a detailed contract that would determine the nature of their obligations and those of their client. The use of a contract to determine the duty of care can avoid the difficulty in applying legal principles observed from an orthodox medicine perspective to the very different environment of complementary medicine.

A contract for services can describe and specify matters such as:

• what services are to be provided, including reference to the nature of the qualifications and training of the practitioner

- what services are not to be provided, such as services expected of a medical practitioner
- the risks of treatment
- a protocol for referral to a medical doctor
- the expected standard of performance of the client, such as attention to diet and exercise regimes
- the nature and extent of the duty of care in regard to that modality
- the cost and length of treatment
- the likely or expected results of treatment
- the susceptibilities and capabilities of the client, and
- the extent to which the practitioner may seek to limit their liability to the client.

This form of contract could avoid misunderstandings and disappointments for both the practitioner and client. It would provide an opportunity for the parties to the contract to specify what considerations are at play in the legal relationship and aspects of the duty of care that will apply. Many complementary medicine practitioners currently obtain from clients a written statement in the form of a questionnaire and a medical history. The contract contemplated above would be much more substantial and would be aimed expressly at specifying the terms of the contract that apply between the parties.

There may be merit in the use of an express contract in circumstances where misunderstandings may arise. This could be effective to protect both the practitioner and client, each of whom may be under some misapprehension about what the other expects from the therapeutic relationship.

In the case of any ambiguity, the courts tend to read such contracts in favour of the client. For this reason, there would have to be clear words to exclude liability for negligence. The provisions of section 60 of the Australian Consumer Law apply a statutory duty for due care and skill that cannot be excluded. The use of an express contract may be vulnerable to common law and statutory claims of undue influence by the practitioner against a powerless client that have the potential to undo such arrangements. This would also be a consideration in regard to whether this is an unfair contract under the Australian Consumer Law discussed at pages 158–159.

This process may be complex for both practitioner and client, and may require the input of lawyers. The expense and complexity of this process may cast doubt on its practicality. This type of contract may not readily be incorporated into the partnership model style of therapeutic relationship contemplated by complementary medicine practitioners if it is intended to aggressively limit or exclude practitioner liability.

Implied contract

More commonly, a contract will arise by implication. When a client seeks professional services from a complementary medicine practitioner, even if no written document is signed, a contract will be created for the provision of those services. This contract will include certain implied terms. There will be an implied contractual obligation between a client and practitioner to use reasonable care and skill, and to provide an explanation of risks of treatment. Accordingly, the content of the obligation based on contract is very similar to the obligation to use reasonable care and skill in the context of an action for negligence.[112] If a client suggests that they have suffered injury because of a lack of reasonable care by the practitioner, they may be entitled to seek redress in contract.

There are some advantages to suing in contract:

- The period of limitation is normally longer than in relation to actions in tort.
- Damages recoverable are not limited to those that are reasonably foreseeable. Damages in contract are based on the loss that flows directly from the alleged breach of contract.

Many professional indemnity insurance policies deny coverage for liability under contract if there would not otherwise have been any liability in tort (discussed on page 227). This could occur when, either by written or oral contract, the practitioner has become contractually bound to produce a particular result, such as the diminution of symptoms, and this has not occurred. Even if the practitioner has been competent in his or her practice, liability could still arise for breach of contract. This provides further incentive to avoid circumstances where liability under a contract could occur.

Health rights complaints legislation

Complementary medicine is acknowledged in all states through health rights complaints statutes.[113] These statutes permit complaints in relation to health professionals, including medical doctors, dentists and a range of health professionals, including complementary medicine practitioners.

Services covered

The statutes make provision for complaints by persons against most health professionals. In almost all cases, the legislation covers virtually all complementary medicine practitioners. This section of the text provides an overview of many significant provisions without undertaking a detailed analysis of each statute in every jurisdiction. Some information requires reference to the specific provisions for each jurisdiction. Specifically incorporated are chiropractors, osteopaths, massage therapists or masseurs, naturopaths, acupuncturists and others in the alternative healthcare or diagnostic fields.[114]

In Western Australia, complementary medicine is probably within the definition of 'health service', which includes a service provided by means of:

a diagnosis or treatment of physical or mental disorder or suspected disorder,
b health care.[115]

Arguably, all therapists not specifically mentioned, such as homoeopaths, would be within the general description of alternative healthcare and diagnostic fields. These statutes grant clients and others the entitlement to bring a complaint against a practitioner. This complaint may result in an investigation of the practices of the healthcare practitioner, and this suggests that some understanding of these statutes is important.

Objects of the legislation

The general scheme common to most statutes will be outlined with reference to the particular features of some individual statutes. Each statute has an object section, preamble or long title that indicates the objectives of the legislation. The following principles or aims are significant in most statutes:

- Improve the quality of provision of health services.
- Provide an accessible and independent regulatory mechanism for the making and resolution of complaints.
- Preserve and promote health rights such as respect for individual dignity, access to adequate information on health services, participation in decision-making and confidentiality of health records.

Complaints

Basis of the complaint

The basis for a complaint is similar in most legislation except New South Wales. In all other states, the grounds for a complaint generally include that a health provider has acted unreasonably:[116]

- in providing the service
- in the manner of providing the service
- in not providing the service
- by denying or restricting access to records
- by not providing information about the user's condition
- by disclosing information in relation to a user
- by failing to exercise due care and skill
- by failing to treat the user in a way that respects a user's needs, wishes and background
- by failing to respect a user's privacy or dignity
- by failing to provide the user with information on treatment or health services available in language the user can understand to allow an informed decision, or on the availability of further advice or relevant education programs, or on the treatment or services received
- by failing to provide the user with reasonable opportunity to make an informed choice of treatment or services available
- by failing to provide the user with a prognosis that it would have been reasonable to provide them
- by acting in disregard of the code or charter of health rights and responsibilities[117]
- as the provision of a health service was not necessary, and as a complaint has been made to the provider but was not properly investigated.

In New South Wales, the basis of the complaint is much narrower. It is limited to:

- the professional conduct of a health practitioner (which would likely encompass many of the above grounds and includes breaches of the *Public Health Act 1991*), and
- a health service that affects the clinical management or care of an individual client.

Notice of complaint

Not surprisingly, a health service provider should be given notice of the complaint made.[118]

Conciliation

An important focus of the health rights complaints statutes is the resolution of complaints by conciliation. In all statutes, after assessment, one option is to refer the matter to conciliation. In New South Wales, the process is voluntary.[119]

The purpose of the conciliation is to resolve the issue and if necessary to enter into enforceable agreements. Normally, a party cannot be represented in the conciliation process unless the conciliator consents as he or she thinks this will assist in the resolution of the dispute.[120] If a resolution is achieved, the commissioner then has the option of not proceeding with the complaint.

If the conciliation does not result in agreement, the matter may be investigated further, referred to a relevant registration body or not proceeded with.[121] It is significant that statements made in conciliation cannot be used outside those proceedings to allow the commencement of an action against a health service provider.[122]

Investigation of complaint

Whether or not the matter proceeds to conciliation, more formal investigations may be made where the relevant minister or the commissioner considers it appropriate.[123] In Victoria, one ground for investigation is whether the complaint is suitable for conciliation.[124] Once an investigation is complete, a report is given to the complainant, the health service provider,[125] if applicable, the relevant registration board, the professional association and the minister.[126] If the report contains an adverse comment about a person, the health professional should be given the opportunity to make comment and lodge a written statement before the report is completed.

Charter of health rights

In some states, there is provision for a code or charter of health rights to be prepared, providing expectations for the performance and obligations of health professionals.[127]

Limitations of provisions

This legislation provides a standard against which a healthcare practitioner can judge the quality of his or her service. By providing principles or objectives in treatment, this legislation can educate and encourage practitioners to consider the purpose of their professional endeavours, which is to provide a service to a client.

Subject to the comments below, the ability to enforce standards of treatment under this legislation is limited because there are no sanctions available for unregistered professions unless there are grounds for referral to the police for criminal matters. The embarrassment and inconvenience of a complaint made against a practitioner may not always be sufficient to improve their performance. For chiropractors, osteopaths and Chinese medicine practitioners, a complaint may generate grounds for disciplinary sanctions including suspension and deregistration by the relevant national registration board pursuant to the National Law and relevant state legislation.

In New South Wales, Queensland, Victoria and South Australia, a complaint may result in unregistered and registered health practitioners (in a matter not relevant to their registration) being subject to a prohibition order or interim prohibition order (refer to page 87).

Application of health complaints statutes

Case study

Mary consults a herbalist, John, about feeling run down. Mary emigrated to Australia recently and has limited English. John is impatient with her language limitations and doesn't mention that she could bring a friend to translate or could access a professional translator. Mary fails to follow John's instructions because she doesn't understand them and doesn't feel comfortable with John. John brusquely tells her to go to someone else.

John's approach does not conform to the principles underlying the health complaints legislation or any health code or charter, which require that practitioners acknowledge the special circumstances of a client. If Mary chooses to complain about John, the relevant body may seek to conciliate the matter after investigation, unless the parties can resolve the matter between themselves. John may be advised about how he could deal with similar situations in the future. As John is not a registered professional, there is no mechanism to bring a claim for professional misconduct to a registration board. The action by the complaints body may start and end with the investigation, conciliation and report. John may be subject to disciplinary procedures by a professional body of which he is a member if Mary complains to that body.

This type of therapeutic relationship demonstrates a lack of trust and open communication. This is conducive to misunderstanding, and increases the chances of a negligence claim being made against the practitioner. A more appropriate response would have included options such as:

- showing a greater degree of understanding and sympathy for Mary's language difficulties
- seeking translation assistance for the client, either through government agencies or through the client's family, while obtaining appropriate release for breach of confidentiality
- writing instructions down for later translation with careful monitoring to ensure understanding, and
- referral to a practitioner with an appropriate language capability.

Case study

A chiropractor, Samantha, greets her new client, Roger. On the previous visit (his first), Samantha had completed an assessment of Roger and had done some very gentle adjustments to his spine. Samantha has indicated that she prefers very gentle forms of manipulation. On this visit, Samantha asks Roger to lie face down on the treatment table. Without explanation, she commences with a dramatic adjustment to his neck and then to his lower back. Roger expresses shock at the nature of the treatment.

Samantha has failed to provide maximum information to a client and does not involve the client in his own care. It would obviously have been advisable to indicate to Roger the nature of the contemplated treatment and to obtain his consent.

A complaint may result in an investigation or conciliation. If deemed appropriate, the matter could be referred to the chiropractors' registration board, either before or after investigation. This board may choose to bring disciplinary proceedings against the practitioner. This behaviour has potential ramifications in terms of the obligation to obtain consent to treatment and to provide warnings about the effect of treatment.

New Zealand provisions

The *Health and Disability Commissioner Act 1994* provides a complaint mechanism for health consumers. Under this legislation, a Health and Disability Commissioner is appointed.[128] Pursuant to section 31 of this legislation, any person may complain orally or in writing to a health and disability services consumer advocate or the commissioner that any action of a healthcare provider appears to be in breach of the Code of Health and Disability Services Consumers' Rights.

A healthcare provider is defined in section 3 to include a 'health practitioner' or 'any other person who provides, or holds himself or herself out as providing, health services to the public or to any section of the public, whether or not any charge is made for those services'. 'Health practitioner' is defined to include a registered health practitioner under the *Health Practitioner Competence Assurance Act 2003*—that is, it would include chiropractors and osteopaths. 'Health services' is defined to include services to promote health or protect health, or to prevent disease or ill-health. Accordingly, this definition would include unregistered complementary medicine practitioners.

The Code of Health and Disability Services Consumers' Rights was finalised in 2007.[129] The Code outlines the rights of consumers, such as to be treated with respect; to be protected from discrimination, coercion, harassment and exploitation; to dignity and independence; to services of an appropriate standard; to effective communication; to be fully informed; to make an informed choice and give informed consent; to support; and to complain.

If a complaint is made to an advocate and the advocate cannot resolve the complaint, it must be referred to the Health and Disability Commissioner. After a preliminary assessment, the commissioner may refer the complaint to an appropriate agency under sections 34 or 36; refer it to an advocate; call a conference; investigate the complaint personally; or decide not to take any action if it is deemed unnecessary or inappropriate. The complaint may be investigated and may involve a referral to the Human Rights Review Tribunal or to a professional body.

Under section 57, damages may be awarded by the Human Rights Review Tribunal, which may declare that the action of the defendant was in breach of the Code; restrain actions in breach of the Code; or order redress or any other relief the tribunal thinks fit. Decisions made pursuant to this legislation provide an insight into how these provisions have been applied in different therapeutic circumstances.[130]

Notes

1   [1932] AC 562 at 580.
2   *Blyth v Birmingham Waterworks* (1856) 11 Ex Ch 781 at 784.
3   *Civil Liability Act 2002* (NSW); *Civil Law (Wrongs) Act 2002* (ACT); *Personal Injuries (Liabilities and Damages) Act 2003* (NT); *Civil Liability Act 2003* (Qld); *Civil Liability Act 1936* (SA); *Wrongs Act 1958* (Vic); *Civil Liability Act 2002* (Tas); *Civil Liability Act 2002* (WA).
4   Stone & Matthews, *Complementary Medicine and the Law*, p. 162; C. Feasby, 'Determining Standard of Care in *Alternative* Contexts' (1997) 5 *Health Law Journal* 46 at 51.
5   Feasby, 'Determining Standard of Care in Alternative Contexts', Ibid.
6   Ibid.
7   Stone & Matthews, *Complementary Medicine and the Law*, p. 168.
8   Exceptions are the Interim Committee for Australian Homoeopathic Standards, *National Competency Standard for Acupuncture* (1999).
9   A. Bensoussan & S. Myers, *Towards a Safer Choice: The Practice of Traditional Chinese Medicine in Australia*, Faculty of Health, University of Western Sydney, Sydney, 1996, Chapter 4.
10 Ibid., pp. 49–75. Refer also to *R v Thomas Sam*; *R v Manju Sam* (No. 18) [2009] NSWSC 1003 (28 September 2009), involving a conviction on a charge of manslaughter involving homoeopathy.
11 Bensoussan & Myers, *Towards a Safer Choice*, p. 81.
12 Ibid., p. 73.
13 Ibid., p. 83.
14 A.M. Kleynhans, 'Complications of and Contraindications to Spinal Manipulative Therapy', in Scott Haldeman (ed.), *Modern Developments in the Principles and Practice of Chiropractic*, Appleton-Century-Crofts, New York, 1980, p. 359; Peter Modde, 'Mal- practice an Inevitable Result of Chiropractic Philosophy and Training' (1979) February *Legal Aspects of Medical Practice* 20.
15 A. Terrett, 'Misuse of the Literature by Medical Authors in Discussing Spinal Manipulative Therapy' (1995) 18 *Journal of Manipulative and Physiological Therapeutics* 4, 203.
16 www.coaghealthcouncil.gov.au/Announcements/ArtMID/527/ArticleID/54/Final-Report-A-National-Code-of-Conduct-for-health-care-workers (accessed 3 November 2021).
17 McIlwraith & Madden, *Health Care and the Law,* 6th ed., Thomson Reuters, Sydney, 2014, p. 198.
18 *Rogers v Whitaker* (1992) 109 ALR 628.
19 R.P. Balkin & J.L.R. Davis, *Law of Torts,* 4th ed., Lexis Nexis Butterworths, Sydney, 2009, p. 268; J.G. Fleming, *The Law of Torts*, Law Book Company, Sydney, 1998, p. 117.
20 *Bolam v Friern Hospital Management Committee* [1957] 1 WLR 582.
21 *Rogers v Whitaker* (1992) 109 ALR 628.
22 *Rogers v Whitaker* (1992) 109 ALR 628.
23 *Yates Property Corporation Pty Ltd (In Liq) and Another v Boland and Ors* (1998) 157 ALR 30 at 51.
24 L. Campbell et al., *Risk Management in Chiropractic: Developing Risk Management Strategies*, Health Services, Fincastle, VA, 1990, p. 31.
25 Balkin & Davis, *Law of Torts,* p. 275; Fleming, *The Law of Torts*, p. 124.
26 Balkin & Davis, *Law of Torts,* p. 277; Fleming, *The Law of Torts*, p. 127.
27 Ibid.
28 *Clark v McLennan* [1983] 1 All ER 416.
29 *Rogers v Whitaker* (1992) 109 ALR 628 at 631.
30 [2005] VSCA 281.
31 *Zhang v Hardas* (No. 2) [2018] NSWSC 432.
32 *Zhang v Hardas* (No. 2) [2018] NSWSC 432 [169]-[170].
33 Stone & Matthews, *Complementary Medicine and the Law*, p. 162.
34 (1987) Australian Torts Reports 80–96.
35 Unreported [1990] SASC (2 July 1990).

36 *Penner v Theobald* (1962) 40 WLR 219; Feasby, 'Determining Standard of Care in Alternative Contexts', at 58.
37 Stone & Matthews, *Complementary Medicine and the Law*, p. 161.
38 *Bennett v Minister of Community Welfare* (1992)176CLR 408; B. Bennett, *Law and Medicine*, Law Book Company, Sydney, 1997, p. 50.
39 *Chappel v Hart* (1998) 156 ALR 517 at 5.
40 [2005] VSCA 281.
41 Stone & Matthews, *Complementary Medicine and the Law*, pp. 169–70.
42 *Chappel v Hart* (1998) 156 ALR 517 at 547.
43 Fleming, *The Law of Torts*, p. 235. 43.
44 (1999, 25 August) NSWCA 306.
45 *Chappel v Hart* (1998) 156 ALR 517 at 548.
46 For example, *Law Reform (Miscellaneous) Provisions Act 1944* (NSW), Pt 2.
47 Feasby, 'Determining Standard of Care in Alternative Contexts', at 1.
48 Stone & Matthews, *Complementary Medicine and the Law*, p. 162.
49 In the United States, the same test is used for osteopathy and naturopathy. Feasby, 'Determining Standard of Care in Alternative Contexts' at 57.
50 *Bawden v Marin* [1990] SASC (2 July 1990).
51 Ibid., at 2.
52 Ibid., at 2.
53 M.H. Cohen, 'Holistic Health Care: Including Alternative and Complementary Medicine in Insurance and Regulatory Schemes' (1996) 38 *Arizona Law Review* 83 at 142.
54 F v R (1983) 33 SASR 189.
55 *Shakoor v Situ* [2000] 4 All ER 181.
56 Ibid.
57 Ibid., at 187.
58 Ibid., at 189.
59 Ibid.
60 Ibid., at 191–192.
61 Stone & Matthews, *Complementary Medicine and the Law*, p. 167. 61.
62 Ibid., p. 168.
63 Ibid., p. 167.
64 Note, however, the facts and decision in Bawden's case, where broken ribs from chiropractic manipulation were deemed not negligent; and Campbell et al., *Risk Management in Chiropractic*, p. 3.
65 *Rosenberg v Rosenberg* 492A. 2d 371 NJ (1985) at 378.
66 Feasby, 'Determining Standard of Care in Alternative Contexts', at 59.
67 Ibid., at 63.
68 *Hardy v Dahl* 187 SE 788 (NC 1936) involved a naturopath who treated a child with diphtheria where a cure was not effected. In *Kirschner v Keller* 42 NE.2d 463 (Ohio Ct App.), a client with epilepsy sought chiropractic treatment and was said to have relied on manipulation to the exclusion of drug treatment. In *Schneider v Revici* 817 F.2d 987 (2d Cir. 1987), a client undertook alternative treatment for breast cancer. In all these cases, voluntary assumption of risk was a successful defence against a negligence claim. See Feasby, 'Determining Standard of Care in Alternative Contexts' at 63–4.
69 *Crossman v Stewart* (1977) 5 CCLT 45.
70 *Schliesman v Fisher* (1979) 158 Cal Rptr 527.
71 Campbell et al., *Risk Management in Chiropractic*, p. 32. 71.
72 Ibid., p. 63.
73 *Law Reform Act 1995* (Qld), s 6.
74 *Green v Walker* (1990) 910 F. 2d 291; *Thomsen v Davison* [1975] Qd R 93. 7.
75 *Magana v Elie* (1982) 439 NE. 2d 1319.
76 A. Grubb, *Principles of Medical Law*, 2nd ed., Oxford University Press, Oxford, 2004, p. 413.
77 *Tabet v Gett* (2010) 84 ALJR 292; 'Tabet v Gett: The End of Loss of Chance Actions in Australia?' (2010) 18 JLM 50

78 *The Australian* (Sydney, Australia), 12 April 2001, 4.
79 'Call For Control on Alternative Medicine', *The Age* (Melbourne), 25 September 2002, 1.
80 *R v Thomas Sam; R v Manju Sam* (No. 18) [2009] NSWSC 1003 (28 September 2009).
81 Quoted in Mostrom v Pettibon 400 S.W.2d 243.
82 *Kerkman v. Hintz* 607P.2d 864.
83 *Chappel v Hart* (1998) 156 ALR 517 at 558, from *F v R* (1983) 33 SASR 189 at 193.
84 (1992) 109 ALR 625.
85 Ibid., at 631.
86 Ibid., at 634.
87 *Chappel v Hart* (1998) 156 ALR 517 at 547.
88 Bensoussan & Myers, *Towards a Safer Choice*, Chapter 4.
89 *Green v Chenoweth* [1998] 2 Qd R 572.
90 Stone & Matthews, *Complementary Medicine and the Law*, p. 170.
91 www.osteopathyboard.gov.au/Codes-Guidelines.aspx
92 *Rogers v Whitaker* (1992) 109 ALR 625 at 634.
93 McIlwraith & Madden, *Health Care and the Law*, p. 278.
94 Stone & Matthews, *Complementary Medicine and the Law*, pp. 175–7.
95 L. Skene, *Law and Medical Practice Rights, Duties, Claims and Defence*, 3rd ed., Lexis Nexis Butterworths, Sydney, 2008, p. 84.
96 Stone & Matthews, *Complementary Medicine and the Law*, p. 173.
97 Ibid.
98 McIlwraith & Madden, *Health Care and the Law*, p. 76.
99 For example, refer to *Minors and Property and Contracts Act 1970* (NSW).
100 McIlwraith & Madden, *Health Care and the Law*, p. 100.
101 Refer also to McIlwraith & Madden, *Health Care and the Law*, Chapter 6.
102 *Minors (Property and Contracts) Act 1970* (NSW), s 49(2); *Consent to Medical Treatment and Palliative Care Act 1995* (SA), s 6—the age when a minor can provide valid consent for medical treatment is sixteen years.
103 (1992) 175 CLR 218 at 238.
104 [1986] AC 112.
105 Ibid., at 188–9.
106 McIlwraith & Madden, *Health Care and the Law*, p. 100.
107 Law Reform Commission of Western Australia, Project no. 77, *Medical Treatment for Minors*, June 1998, p. 6. 36.
108 Stone & Matthews, *Complementary Medicine and the Law*, p. 182.
109 Ibid., p. 181.
110 Skene, *Law and Medical Practice Rights*, p. 46.
111 Many codes of conduct prohibit advertising of cures by practitioners. It is a moot point whether this type of regulation might be deemed to be anti-competitive in nature and invalid.
112 Skene, *Law and Medical Practice Rights*, p. 47.
113 *Health Care Complaints Act 1993* (NSW); (Vic.); *Health Ombudsman Act 2013* (Qld); *Health and Disability Services (Complaints) Act 1995* (WA); *Health Complaints Act 1995* (Tas); *Health and Community Services Complaints Act 2004* (SA); *Human Rights Commission Act 2005* (ACT); *Health and Community Services Complaints Act 1998* (NT).
114 NSW, s 4; Vic, s 3; Qld, ss 7, 8; SA, s 4; Tas, s 3, Part 1, Schedule 1; NT, s 4; ACT, s 74, Part 1, schedule 2 regulations.
115 *Health and Disability Services (Complaints) Act 1995* (WA), s 3
116 Vic, s 5; Qld, s 31; WA, s 25; Tas, s 23; SA, s 25; ACT, s 22; NT, s 23.
117 Tas, s 23(1)(k); NT, s 23(1)(k).
118 NSW, ss 16, 28; Qld, ss 35, 70; Tas, s 27; WA, s 33; SA s 55; ACT, s 45.
119 Section 48 of NSW Act.
120 NSW, s 50; Vic, no mention of this issue; Qld, no mention of this issue; WA, s 39(1); Tas, s 33; SA, s 37; ACT, s 58; NT, s 40.
121 Vic, s 44; Qld, ss 147,148.
122 Vic, s 43(14)(15); Qld, s 150; WA, s 42; Tas, s 37; SA, s 40; NT, s 47.
123 Qld, s 148; Vic, s 45; Tas, s 40(1)(2); WA, s 45; NT, s 20, s 48(1).

124 Section 37.
125 NSW, s 40; Qld, s 145; SA, s 55.
126 NSW, ss 39, 41, 42; SA, ss 54, 55; Tas, s 55; ACT, s 83; NT, if applicable the Speaker, s 65(2) (a).
127 Tasmania, Part 3; ACT, Part VI; NT, s 104; ACT and Qld, Code of Health Rights and Responsibilities; SA, Charter of Health and Community Services Rights; Tas, Charter of Health Rights; NT, Code of Health and Community Rights and Responsibilities.
128 *Health and Disability Commissioner Act 1994*, s 8 (NZ).
129 Code of Health and Disability Services Consumers' Rights Regulations 1996.
130 Director of Proceedings (Health and Disability) and A, Decision no. 35/03 HRRT 15/02; The Director of Health and Disability Proceedings and DG, Decision no. 2/05, ref. no. HRRT 22/04; The Director of Health and Disability Proceedings and DG, Decision no 3/05, ref. no. HRRT 23/04.

6 Goods and consumer issues

As well as supplying services, many practitioners supply substances such as vitamins, food supplements and herbs to their clients. The Commonwealth government seeks to ensure that these substances are not harmful to users, are manufactured properly, perform as represented and are advertised in a way that does not mislead the users. The *Therapeutic Goods Act 1989* (Cth) ('TGA') or state equivalents apply to many of these substances. Many complementary medicine professional activities are exempt from this legislation if certain criteria apply, but it is vital for the practitioner to know what these criteria are in order to stay within the law. This chapter provides a general overview of some of the provisions likely to be relevant to complementary medicine practitioners. As the TGA is complex and very specific in relation to how it may impact on particular substances and practices, practitioners should seek independent legal advice on any matters that apply directly to their practice.

This chapter also deals with consumer legislation such as the *Sale of Goods Acts*, *Competition and Consumer Act 2010* and *Fair Trading Acts*, which affect the way a practitioner may market and advertise their goods and services. Like any business, practitioners need to avoid representations that are false, misleading or deceptive to their clients. In addition this chapter will briefly deal with the provisions of the national Australian Consumer Law, which may impact upon the enforceability of consumer contracts entered into by complementary medicine practitioners where the terms of that contract could be seen as unfair.

BOX 6.1

Action plan

- Understand the basic scheme of the *Therapeutic Goods Act* (TGA).
- If prescribing therapeutic substances from another manufacturer such as vitamins or herbs ensure the substances are either listed or registered under the TGA.
- If you are not exempt from the registration or listing requirements of the TGA, seek legal advice.
- If you manufacture therapeutic goods, make sure you or your product are exempt from the manufacturing provisions of the TGA.
- If you are not exempt from the manufacturing provisions of the TGA, seek legal advice.
- Label your therapeutic goods clearly and in accordance with legal requirements.
- Make sure that the marketing and advertising of your services and goods comply with the TGA.

DOI: 10.4324/9781003195931-6

Therapeutic Goods Act 1989

The TGA and the equivalent statutes for New South Wales, Victoria, Queensland, South Australia and Tasmania, and in the Territories, regulate the use of therapeutic goods in complementary medicine.[1] In these jurisdictions, the TGA applies with full force as if it were a statute passed by those state or territory governments subject to some local provisions, while the coverage of the TGA is more limited in Western Australia.

Understanding the basic scheme of the Therapeutic Goods Act

Types of goods covered

Therapeutic goods are defined in section 3 of the TGA to include goods that are represented in any way to be, or that are—whether because of the way in which the goods are presented or for any other reason—likely to be taken to be for therapeutic use, or used as an ingredient or component in the manufacture of therapeutic goods or for use as a container for goods. This definition could include therapeutic goods that do not make therapeutic claims when there is a representation that the goods are for therapeutic use. The TGA itself does not specifically define complementary medicine though there is a definition under the Therapeutic Goods Regulation 1990, section 2, discussed below, for specified purposes.

'Therapeutic use' is defined widely in section 3 to include use in preventing, diagnosing, curing or alleviating a disease, ailment, defect or injury in persons, or influencing, inhibiting or modifying a physiological process in persons.

The TGA controls the supply, import, export, manufacture and advertising of goods that are, or are represented as likely to be, for therapeutic use. This covers most of the substances, herbs and remedies used by complementary medicine practitioners. To determine whether your practices or business are regulated by the TGA, consider the following steps.

Step 1: Practitioners not subject to TGA

If you *do not* supply to clients any herbs, vitamins, nutritional substances, homoeopathic remedies, drugs or other therapeutic goods or therapeutic devices, then the TGA does not affect you. If you *do* supply these types of goods, this discussion is relevant.

BOX 6.2

Practice tip

If you recommend that a client should purchase and use a substance such as a homoeopathic remedy or vitamins, but play no part in its supply or manufacture, the TGA would not apply to that transaction, though the party who manufactures or supplies this product may be subject to the TGA.

Object of legislation

The object of the TGA is to create a national scheme consisting of controls provided by the TGA and complementary state legislation. A national scheme is necessary because, under the federal Constitution, the Commonwealth has a limited ability to pass laws on therapeutic goods. The Commonwealth has power to legislate with regard to the activities of a corporation related to trade and commerce across state or national borders or in relation to providing pharmaceutical or repatriation benefits and in regard to the territories.[2] State legislation plugs the gaps in the scheme for things done *within* a state. To date, only Western Australia has not passed legislation that applies the provisions of the Commonwealth legislation at the state level.

The limited constitutional powers of the Commonwealth impact on the effectiveness of the TGA in Western Australia. For example, a practitioner who prepares a homoeopathic treatment or prescribes a herb in Western Australia is not affected by the TGA if the transaction has no international or interstate aspect.[3] As a result it is likely many transactions of a homoeopath, herbalist or traditional Chinese medicine practitioner in Western Australia would not be caught by the TGA. For practitioners within the territories, New South Wales, Victoria, Queensland, South Australia and Tasmania, the Commonwealth and mirror state and territory legislation will apply to all of those activities.

The objects of the TGA are supported by the licensing and auditing of manufacturers of complementary medicines, including the application of the *Guide to Good Manufacturing Practice for Medicinal Products*, pre-market assessment of complementary medicines and post-market activities involving audits and testing of products. The Therapeutic Goods Administration administers the legislation.

The role of the Advisory Committee on Complementary Medicines

An Advisory Committee on Complementary Medicines (ACCM) evaluates and reports on the registration or listing of complementary medicines. Complementary medicines are specifically defined under the Therapeutic Goods Regulation section 2 and would be considered to be therapeutic goods based upon the definition of that term. For the purpose of the establishment and membership of the ACCM and for issues relevant to listing and exemptions associated with complementary medicine, it is defined in the Therapeutic Goods Regulation section 2 as therapeutic goods 'consisting wholly or principally of one or more designated active ingredients, each of which has a clearly established identity and a traditional use'. The type of complementary medicine product includes traditional medicines, herbal medicines; homoeopathic medicines; anthroposophic medicines; essential oils and nutritional supplements.[4]

The Therapeutic Goods Regulation section 2 defines 'designated active ingredients' based upon Schedule 14 of the regulations as including substances such as essential oils, herbal substances, plant fibres and chlorophyll, homoeopathic preparations, vitamins or royal jelly. 'Traditional use' is defined by the Therapeutic Goods Regulation section 2 to refer to the use of a designated active ingredient that is well documented according to the accumulated experience of many traditional healthcare practitioners over an extended period of time and that accords with well-established procedures of preparation, application and dosage.

Standards

Chapter 3 section 10 of the TGA allows the minister to publish a standard for particular therapeutic goods that sets minimum requirements for matters such as quantity in containers, quality and manufacturing process. A person must not import, export or supply therapeutic goods without consent under the TGA if they do not conform to a standard applicable to the goods. If harm has or will result, possible both civil and criminal offences may arise.[5]

Complementary medicine practitioners are not exempt from these provisions. Currently, there are no standards for raw Chinese herbs.[6] This means that a person can import or supply raw Chinese herbs without complying with a standard. There may be an applicable standard for other substances, such as herbs based on the British Pharmacopoeia and/or a Therapeutic Goods Order under the TGA.

Part 3: Australian Register of Therapeutic Goods

Part 3-2 Division 1 of the TGA prescribes a number of criminal and civil offences in relation to therapeutic goods for use in humans. These offences include the import, export, manufacture or supply of therapeutic goods unless they are registered or listed goods *in relation to the person*, are exempt goods or the TGA otherwise permits it. Similar provisions in relation to wholesale supply are found in section 21. There are general offences in sections 22-22 B in regard to purported registration or listing numbers; false advertising of therapeutic goods indications; a breach of a condition of exempt goods if it is likely to cause serious risk to public health, or false or misleading statements in regard of registration of therapeutic goods.

Note that registered or listed goods must be registered or listed in relation to a specific party. This means that a party would need to apply for registration or listing as discussed below in relation to a specific product, and obtain approval from the Therapeutic Goods Administration if they intend to legally import, export, manufacture or supply the therapeutic good.

Obtaining registration or listing of therapeutic goods used in practice is probably beyond the resources of most practitioners. Unless a practitioner can demonstrate that they are dealing with exempt goods or that they are exempt from the provisions of the TGA, they will be in breach of this provision when they import, export, manufacture or supply therapeutic goods without being listed or registered in relation to those goods.

The provisions of Chapter 2 of the TGA require the secretary of the relevant department to establish an Australian Register of Therapeutic Goods for compiling information in relation to therapeutic goods and their evaluation for use in humans. The register contains registered goods and listed goods. The registration or listing of goods requires an application to be made under section 23 and payment of the applicable fee.

- *Registered goods.* Registration involves an exhaustive appraisal of the quality, safety and efficacy of the goods for the purpose intended from controlled clinical trials or if available from other well-accepted sources such as standard textbooks. Registration is necessary for substances considered high risk, and includes all prescription medicines containing ingredients included in Schedule 4 or Schedule 8 of the Standard for the Uniform Scheduling of Drugs and Poisons. Some low-risk, non-prescription drugs may be registered if it is considered necessary to ensure adequate labelling for safe use. Registered goods are also assessed for presentation, conformity with an applicable standard and appropriateness of manufacturing process. For complementary medicines, the ACCM provides expertise to the relevant department in relation to registration. Some complementary medicines are registered. Registered products can be recognised by the notation 'AUST R No xxx' shown on the label.

*   *Listed goods.* These are goods with a perceived lower risk, usually self-selected by consumers and used for self-treatment. Listing involves a low-cost, streamlined electronic process for assessment of the quality, safety, presentation, manufacturing process and conformity with standards. Listing does not require scientific justification of claims made, though a person who has listed goods may be asked to provide evidence of the formulation, composition, methods of manufacture and safety of the goods, and evidence or information to support any therapeutic claims made.[7] Most complementary medicines are listed substances. Listed substances are identified by the 'AUST L No xxx' notation on the label. Another new type of listed medicine, 'assessed listed medicine', allows more substantial indications as the TGA has assessed the evidence of the sponsor for the medicine's indications. Other listed medicines rely upon self-certification.[8] Medicines through the assessed listed medicines pathway will be included in the ARTG following self-certification of the safety and quality of the product, and TGA pre-market assessment of efficacy evidence supporting the proposed indications.[9]

Most practitioners will not wish to be involved in listing or registering their own substances, and will purchase substances from suppliers who will have obtained either registration or listing for the substance. Both listed and registered goods are required to be manufactured pursuant to the *Guide to Good Manufacturing Practice for Medicinal Products*, and may be subject to the need for advisory or warning labels. There is a list of substances that may be used as active ingredients in listed medicines on the TGA. Refer to Part 1, Schedule 4 of the Regulations, which specifies substances including some complementary medicines that should be included in the register as listed goods.

The Australian Regulatory Guidelines for Listed Medicines and Registered Complementary Medicines[10] provide guidance about how sponsors of complementary medicines can satisfy the requirements to list or register complementary medicine under the TGA.

Practitioner only products

Provision is made in the regulatory regime for what are called 'For Practitioner Dispensing Only' products. This allows a listed or registered complementary medicine to be supplied in a dispensing pack to a registered complementary healthcare practitioner (the requirement for registration would appear to limit this provision to osteopaths, chiropractors and Chinese medicine practitioners, though in practice this limitation is not normally applied and it seems commonly non-registered complementary healthcare practitioners such as Western herbal medicine and naturopaths also enjoy this dispensation—refer to the discussion below). The dispensing pack should be labelled 'For Practitioner Dispensing Only'. These medicines must meet the standards of other listed or registered complementary medicines but they do not need to include a statement of their purpose/therapeutic indication of the therapeutic good on the label. Refer to section 8(n) of Therapeutic Goods Order no. 92 (General Requirements for Labels for Medicines) in relation to this requirement. The intention is that these medicines will be supplied after a consultation between the practitioner and the consumer, with the practitioner attaching a label providing instructions for use for the client.

Are you exempt from the need to register or list the product?

Step 2

If you are involved in the supply, export, import or manufacturing of therapeutic goods, you are subject to the Part 3 requirements for registration or listing, unless exempt from the TGA. You will need specific legal advice to determine your status. Read this section for some general comments about whether you could be exempt.

Practitioners may be able to take advantage of the substantial exemptions from many provisions of the TGA. Schedule 5 of the Regulations describes therapeutic goods exempt from the operation of Part 3-2 of the TGA—that is, they do not require registration or listing and can be imported, exported and supplied either by retail or wholesale. The exemptions likely to be relevant to complementary medicine practitioners include therapeutic goods that are:

* homoeopathic preparations[11] that do not include ingredients of an animal or human origin, more dilute than a one thousand-fold dilution of a mother tincture, and which are not required to be sterile
* starting materials (this term is not defined but would likely include raw Chinese herbs used in the manufacture of therapeutic goods, except when pre-packaged for supply for other therapeutic purposes or formulated as a dosage form), and
* medicines that are dispensed or extemporaneously compounded for a particular person for therapeutic application to that person. This would probably apply to herbal substances or homoeopathic preparations (not exempt as above) dispensed to clients after a consultation or compounded at the time of a consultation.

If these exemptions do not apply, or if you are uncertain about whether or not they do, seek legal advice because the requirements of the statute in relation to registration and listing of therapeutic goods may apply to your practice.

BOX 6.3

Practice tip

A breach of the TGA may occur due to non-compliance with the limitations of the relevant exemptions. This might occur where a practitioner attempts to sell, from a health food store, herbal substances that are pre-packaged for supply or homoeopathic mixtures that are not exempt as not sufficiently dilute, and they are not dispensed or compounded for a particular person but simply placed on sale for any person to purchase. If you dispense a pre-prepared vitamin tonic that does not contain a substance that requires listing or registration to a client as part of your practice as a naturopath, you do not need to list this substance and are entitled to supply it to a client if it is dispensed as part of a consultation.

Manufacturing of therapeutic goods Part 3–3

Step 3

If you sell registered or listed therapeutic goods that are entirely pre-prepared by the party legally entitled to wholesale those products, then the provisions of Part 3–3 may not be applicable. If you are involved in any activity that might be manufacturing, including preparing, assembling or packaging, then Part 3–3 may apply to you. Once again, most complementary medicine practitioners will seek exemption from this part. Read this section to ascertain what factors determine whether you and your product are exempt. You will require specific legal advice to determine your status.

The term 'manufacture' is defined widely in section 3 of the TGA to include a person producing goods or engaging in any part of the process of producing the goods or bringing the goods to their final state, such as processing, assembling, packaging, labelling, storing, sterilising, testing or releasing for supply. This would include the processes of preparation involved in, for example, the preparation of herbs or the final preparation of homoeopathic medicine for a client from a mother tincture. Unless exempted, a manufacturer of medicinal products must comply with the *Guide to Good Manufacturing Practice for Medicinal Products*, which is based upon an international standard.

Sections 35 and 35A provide for criminal and civil liability if a person carries out a step in the manufacture of therapeutic goods for supply for use in humans at premises in Australia unless:

- the goods are exempt, or
- the person is exempt in relation to the manufacture of the goods, or
- the person is the holder of a licence that authorises the carrying out of a step in relation to the goods at those premises.

This potentially makes many activities of complementary medicine practitioners an offence of manufacturing without a licence under the TGA. The concern is avoided if either the practitioner or the goods can be deemed exempt from the legislation. Fortunately, many goods and activities are exempt.

Are you or your goods exempt from the manufacturing requirements of the TGA?

Exempt goods

Schedule 7 of the regulations exempts some therapeutic goods from the provisions of Part 3-3 of the TGA. So far as is relevant for complementary medicine practitioners, this could relate to:

- ingredients, except water, used in the manufacture of therapeutic goods where the ingredients do not have a therapeutic action or are herbs, bulk hamamelis or oils extracted from herbs, the sole therapeutic use of which is as starting materials for use by licensed manufacturers, and

- homoeopathic preparations more dilute than a one thousand-fold dilution of a mother tincture and that are not required to be sterile.

Exempt persons

Of even more importance is Schedule 8 of the regulations, which exempts particular persons from the operation of Part 3-3 of the Act. These include herbalists, nutritionists, naturopaths, practitioners of traditional Chinese medicine or homoeopathic practitioners engaged in the manufacture of any herbal, homoeopathic or nutritional supplement preparation, where:

- the preparation is for use in the course of his or her business, and
- the preparations are manufactured on premises that the person carrying on the business occupies and that he or she is able to close so as to exclude the public, and
- the person carrying on the business supplies the preparation for administration to a particular person after consulting with that person and uses his or her own judgement as to the treatment required.

Accordingly, within the parameters of this exemption, there is no obligation on a practitioner to comply with the requirements of Part 3-3 of the TGA, which requires the obtaining of a licence to manufacture therapeutic goods.

Step 4

If your practice is not exempt from the manufacturing provisions or you are uncertain, seek legal advice.

BOX 6.4

Practice tip

A breach of the TGA may occur if the substance was manufactured by the practitioner and is included as part of the stock at a health shop associated with the practice, such that it could not be said it was supplied after consultation with the client based on the therapist's judgement.

Labelling and promotion under the TGA

The *Therapeutic Goods Act* regulates medicines in Australia that include the requirements for labelling of substances including product name, batch number, storage conditions and directions for use.[12] The *Therapeutic Goods Order No. 92—Standard for labels of non-prescription medicines* includes provisions that may exempt complementary medicine practitioners from these requirements.

BOX 6.5

Practice tip

Even if exempted, practitioners should voluntarily comply with the labelling require-ments in order to provide maximum information to the client and thereby encourage accurate and safe use of prescribed substances.

Clause 5(1)(m) states that this Order does not apply to a medicine that is:

> made up or compounded extemporaneously, for a specific and individual case, by a complementary healthcare practitioner in the lawful practice of his or her profession.

The term 'complementary healthcare practitioner' requires reference to section 42 AA(1)(c) of the *Therapeutic Goods Act 1989* which states that term means 'herbalists, homoeopathic practitioners, naturopaths, nutritionists, practitioners of traditional Chinese medicine or podiatrists registered under a law of a State or Territory'.

This should be interpreted to mean that the specified complementary medicine prac-titioners are exempt from this Order. It would in any event suggest that any extempo-raneous medicines should be properly labelled for the client to understand the nature of the substance; dosing and required warnings and directions for use.

Food/medicine interface

Sometimes it may be difficult to determine whether a substance is a food or a ther-apeutic good, especially when the substance makes a health claim. Note that ther-apeutic goods do not usually include goods that have a prescribed standard in the Australia New Zealand Food Standards Code as defined by the *Food Standards Australia New Zealand Act 1991* (Cth) or goods that have a tradition in Australia and New Zealand for use as foods for humans in the form in which they are presented. These foods should not be marketed as having therapeutic properties. If a substance is a food it will be regulated by state and Commonwealth food quality regulators. If a product is taken orally and is not covered by the TGA it is likely to be regulated as a food.

A Food/Medicine Interface Guidance Tool is available to determine which category a substance falls into by asking seven questions. This tool is available on the TGA website at https://www.tga.gov.au/food-medicine-interface-guidance-tool-fmigt.

Under section 7 of the TGA, it is possible for some substances that might appear to be a food to be declared to be a therapeutic good.

These goods are subject to the requirement to be listed or registered on the Australian Register of Therapeutic Goods.

The practitioner should be concerned that, if the TGA provisions have been ignored, there has been no assessment or review process to at least partly ensure the quality and efficacy of the product.

BOX 6.6

Practice tip

If a practitioner is supplying a substance such as a herb or homoeopathic substance manufactured by another, the criteria relevant for the exemption of that substance from the provisions of the TGA discussed above may not be present. In that case, the product should have on the label a notation of the registration or listing number under the TGA. If the registration or listing number is not shown, then perhaps the substance:

- is not a therapeutic good (it may be a food), or
- is deemed by the TGA or regulations as exempt from the registration and listing requirements (relevant for some homoeopathic substances), or
- is registered or listed but mislabelled, or
- has been manufactured, supplied or imported in breach of the TGA or state equivalents.

Australian native and endangered species in therapeutic goods

The Australian government is active in regulating the international movement (including import and export) of native fauna and flora under the *Environment Protection and Biodiversity Conservation Act 1999* (Cth) (EPBC). It is also supportive of the efforts of other countries to protect their own fauna and flora that have been identified as significant under the Convention on International Trade in Endangered Species of Wild Fauna and Flora (CITES). These measures may impact on complementary medicine practitioners, such as TCM practitioners, herbalists or naturopaths, who prepare, export or import protected flora or fauna for therapeutic use.

Under Part 13A of the EPBC, the international movement of wildlife and products is controlled. Section 303CA of the EPBC requires the Environment Minister to publish a list of CITES species for the purposes of this Act. This list contains a large number of species of animals and plants that are deemed important to protect. The import or export of such fauna and flora is not permitted unless done with a permit under the EPBC. For this reason, reference to the relevant state Environmental Protection Authorities may be necessary for the trade of Australian native or endangered species or products within Australia. In relation to export or import of this flora or fauna, reference should be made to the Australian Government Department of Agriculture, Water and the Environment at www.environment.gov.au to ensure that these requirements are satisfied.

New Zealand therapeutic goods legislation

Dietary supplements

In New Zealand, many complementary medicines marketed as dietary supplements do not involve pre-market approval processes to determine their efficacy or safety, and to control quality. Dietary supplements are regulated by the Dietary Supplements Regulations 1985. Regulation 2A defines 'dietary supplement' as follows:

1 In these regulations, dietary supplement means something to which subclauses (2) to (6) apply.
2 It is an amino acid, edible substance, herb, mineral, synthetic nutrient or vitamin.
3 It is sold by itself or in a mixture.
4 It is sold in a controlled dosage form as a liquid, powder, or tablet (which might be described on the label as a cachet, capsule, lozenge, or pastille instead of as a tablet).
5 It is intended to be ingested orally.
6 It is intended to supplement the amount of the amino acid, edible substance, herb, mineral, synthetic nutrient, or vitamin normally derived from food.

These regulations contain labelling requirements in Regulations 4–10. In addition, Regulation 11 confirms that dietary supplements must not make therapeutic claims unless permitted under the *Medicines Act 1981*, discussed below. The explanatory note with the regulations indicates that:

> These regulations, in a sense, fill the gap between the *Food Regulations 2015* and the *Medicines Regulations 1984*, in that dietary supplements are not food or medicine in the ordinary sense of those words. However, they are food within the meaning of the *Food Act 1981*, and will be related products within the meaning of the *Medicines Act 1981* if therapeutic claims are made for them.

Therapeutic goods

The primary legislation in this area is the *Medicines Act 1981*. 'Medicine' is defined in section 3 to include

> any substance or article, other than a medical device, that is manufactured, imported, sold or supplied wholly or principally for administering to one or more human beings for a therapeutic purpose and achieves, or is likely to achieve, its principal intended action in or on the human body by pharmacological, immunological, or metabolic means.

'Therapeutic purpose' is defined in section 4 to include treating or preventing disease.

Manufacture and sale of medicines

Under section 17, no person shall in the course of a business manufacture, sell by wholesale, pack or label a medicine or operate any pharmacy otherwise than pursuant to a licence issued under Part 3 of the *Medicines Act*, subject to sections 25–34 and relevant regulations. Section 17 would regulate some transactions by complementary medicine practitioners in the provision of medicines to clients but for the exemptions discussed below.

Under section 28, there is a significant exemption in relation to dealing with herbal medicines in relation to contemporaneous dispensing after a consultation and subject to some labelling limitations. Section 28 confirms that any person may in the course of a business carried on by that person manufacture, pack and label, or sell or supply, any herbal remedy for administration to a particular person after being requested by or on behalf of that person to use their own judgement as to the treatment required.

Section 28(2) permits a person to manufacture, pack, sell or supply and label any herbal remedy if the substance is sold or supplied under a designation that specifies only the plant from which it is made and the process to which the plant has been subjected during the production of the remedy, and does not apply any other name to the remedy or any written recommendation as to the use of the remedy. 'Herbal remedy' is defined in section 2 as:

> a medicine (not being or containing a prescription medicine, or a restricted medicine, or a pharmacy-only medicine) consisting of—
>
> a   Any substance produced by subjecting a plant to drying, crushing, or any other similar process; or
> b   A mixture comprising 2 or more such substances only; or
> c   A mixture comprising 1 or more such substances with water or ethyl alcohol or any inert substance.

The most significant exemption is section 32, which states:

> Notwithstanding sections 17 and 20 to 24 of this Act or anything in any licence, but subject to the other provisions of this Act and to any regulations made under this Act, any natural therapist or other person may manufacture, pack, label, sell by retail, or supply in circumstances corresponding to retail sale, any medicine that neither is nor contains—
>
> a   A prescription medicine; or
> b   A restricted medicine; or
> c   A pharmacy only medicine—

for administration to a particular person after being requested by or on behalf of that person to use his own judgement as to the treatment required.

This allows a natural therapist (not defined by the legislation) to avoid many of the regulatory requirements of the legislation if the medicine is provided after a consultation. This exemption would relate to what is generally known as a general sales medicine that does not include an ingredient scheduled under the *Misuse of Drugs Act 1975* and that is not one of the other medicines quoted in section 32.

The term 'consultation' is not defined under the legislation; however, there is an expectation that a consultation should involve a genuine dialogue between the natural therapist and the client to ascertain that client's condition in order to suggest what might be an appropriate treatment.

Note that under section 44 there are legal requirements in relation to the packaging used for medicines, including an ability to reseal, being impervious to medicine and being properly labelled.

A useful overview of these provisions is found in the New Zealand Medicines and Medical Devices Safety Authority Information for Health Professionals—Compliance with the *Medicines Act 1981*: Guidance for Natural Health Professionals, www.medsafe.govt.nz/profs/NaturalHealth.asp.[13] This document provides a useful discussion of 'What Natural Therapists can do when operating under the section 32 exemption' and 'What Natural Therapists can't do' and examples of how the provisions apply.

It should be noted that the exemptions provided under this legislation do not allow natural therapists to advertise unapproved general sales medicines. This means that natural therapists may not display products that are labelled to state or imply a therapeutic purpose unless they are approved medicines. In addition, it is not legal to advertise medicines or methods of treatment for the list of ailments in Schedule 1 to the *Medicines Act 1981*. This list includes cancer, diabetes, pneumonia and sexual impotence. Natural therapists are not entitled to advertise that a medicine, treatment or therapeutic device is infallible or a panacea. Natural therapists may advertise that they treat certain conditions but are not entitled to advertise that they specialise in treatment of a specific condition using a named product.

Consumer legislation

Like any business, complementary medicine practitioners in Australia are subject to consumer legislation that imposes obligations on the practitioner as to how goods and services are advertised and supplied. The most important statutes are:

- the *Sale of Goods Act* (SGA) (almost identical provisions in all states)
- the *Commonwealth Competition and Consumer Act 2010* (CCA) and the *Fair Trading Act* (FTA) (similar provisions in all states).

The CCA includes the Australian Consumer Law (ACL), which applies across all jurisdictions in Australia. The *ACCC, Advertising and Selling Guide: A Guide for Business March 2021* provides good information in this area.[14]

Reference will be made to provisions of the ACL in this treatment. This area of law is very complex, and a complete treatment is beyond the scope of this book. This discussion will include some significant issues that may arise for a complementary medicine practitioner. The *Sale of Goods Act* (SGA) applies to any sale of goods, whether involving a consumer or not, and is not affected by the ACL. The ACL applies to transactions involving a consumer.

Sale of Goods Act

What are goods?

Goods are defined to include most items and substances sold by practitioners.[15]

BOX 6.7

Action plan

- Understand your obligations under the Sale of Goods Act when selling products.
- Make sure that, if you describe a product to a client, it satisfies this description.
- Make sure that, if you sell a product for a particular purpose, it is suitable for that purpose.
- Make sure that any product sold is of merchantable quality.

Many complementary medicine practitioners sell goods such as homoeopathic remedies, herbal mixtures or herbs, vitamins, massage oils and equipment. These sales are subject to the SGA legislation in each state.

Sale by description

Where a buyer purchases goods based on a description, there is an implied condition that the goods shall correspond to the description.

If the goods don't fit that description, the purchaser can terminate the contract—that is, return the goods and recover the money they have paid and/or seek damages for any loss incurred. If a herbal mixture, vitamin supplement or massage oil is represented as containing particular ingredients and it doesn't, then the provision would be breached.

Implied condition as to quality or fitness for purpose

The goods should work in the way the buyer has been told they work. There is an implied condition that goods will be reasonably fit for the purpose where:

- the buyer expressly or by implication makes known the purpose to which the goods will be put
- the buyer relies on the vendor's skill and judgement, and
- the goods are in the course of the vendor's business to supply.

The requirement that the buyer makes known the purpose for the goods may not be important where the use contemplated is the ordinary use of the goods. If an unusual use is contemplated, liability for the vendor may not arise unless the intended purpose is revealed expressly to the vendor.

If massage oil is sold and it is not suitable for that purpose, this provision may be breached. A proviso to this section avoids liability when the purchase is made under a trade name where it is obvious that the purchaser did not rely on the vendor's skill and judgement.

Merchantable quality

The goods should be useful for the purpose for which they were bought. Where goods are purchased by description from a vendor who deals in goods of that description (whether the seller is the manufacturer or not), there is an implied condition that the goods are of merchantable quality. 'Merchantable quality' means that goods are commercially saleable for the purpose for which they are normally used. For example, substances such as herbs sold by a practitioner should be fresh (if this is necessary for their potency). This provision does not apply to defects that examination ought to have revealed. These provisions apply whether the vendor was negligent or not, and even if the defects were not obvious to the vendor of the goods.

If massage oil sold is not of merchantable quality because of the manufacturing process, the vendor may be liable even if the defect was not obvious. The manufacturer may also be liable on the basis of manufacturer's liability (see pages 162–163).

Exclusion of implied conditions

The provisions of the SGA may be negated or varied by express agreement or by implication, or based on a course of dealing between the parties. This means that there may be some merit in practitioners considering express exclusions in relation to the provisions of the SGA where these provisions may expose the practitioner unduly. This is only likely to be practical where the contract for sale of goods is substantial enough to justify a written contract. In many states, the ability to exclude these provisions is limited by legislation.

The Australian Consumer Law (ACL)

BOX 6.8

Action plan

- Honest, open, responsible and fair business practices, the hallmarks of professional behaviour, will usually protect against claims under the ACL.
- Put in place standard procedures that ensure compliance with your obligations under the ACL.
- Make sure that, from the point of view of a client, your professional practices are not deceptive or misleading.
- Do not use your influence over a vulnerable client and thereby become involved in unconscionable conduct.
- Make sure your products, services and advice to clients are honest and open, avoiding any false representations as to the need for your services or the quality, standard or performance of the products or services you might provide.

The ACL implies similar (though not identical) guarantees in relation to the supply of goods to a consumer, requiring that those goods are of an acceptable quality, and correspond to description and fitness for purpose.[16] A person acquires goods as a consumer if the goods are for personal, domestic or household use or consumption, and not for the purpose of resale or as part of a manufacturing process.[17]

In addition, the provisions of section 60 imply a warranty that services provided to a consumer will be rendered with due care and skill, and that the services will be reasonably fit for the purpose for which they are supplied. This could apply to the provision of professional services. This liability may overlap with liability in relation to negligence discussed in Chapter 4. If professional negligence claims are made more difficult by the civil liability legislation discussed above, actions under the ACL may become more common. The types of activities that may breach the ACL relate to the following.

Misleading or deceptive behaviour

Don't tell clients things that may not be true or attempt to trick them. The ACL provides that: 'A person shall not, in trade or commerce, engage in conduct that is misleading or deceptive or is likely to mislead or deceive.' This is a very broad provision that covers many specific circumstances dealt with under other sections.

A breach of this provision might include exaggerated claims of the effect of services, such as 100 per cent cures for conditions like back pain or miracle slimming techniques where the claims are not verifiable. Another example is unjustified claims made about the curative effects of certain herbal and homoeopathic substances sold by practitioners.

Unconscionable conduct

Do not take advantage of a vulnerable client. This is fundamental to appropriate professional practice and is reflected in the ACL provision that 'a supplier shall not, in trade or commerce, in connection with the supply or possible supply of goods or services to a person ("the customer"), engage in conduct that is, in all the circumstances, unconscionable'.

The provision describes examples of unconscionable conduct, such as the use of unequal bargaining power or where undue influence or unfair tactics were used in connection with the supply of goods or services. Liability might arise if a client under a disability, such as inexperience or limited English or understanding, was convinced to undertake a course of treatment or to purchase goods in circumstances where the practitioner used his or her position as a health professional to unfairly influence this transaction.

False representations

Goods and services should be what you say they are. The ACL provides that a person shall not, in trade or commerce in connection with the supply or possible supply of goods or services or in connection with the promotion by any means of the supply or use of goods or services, make representations such as:

* falsely representing that goods are of a particular standard, quality, value, grade, composition, style or model or have had a particular history or particular previous use
* falsely representing that services are of a particular standard, quality, value or grade
* falsely representing that goods or services have sponsorship, approval, performance characteristics, accessories, uses or benefits they do not have, and
* making a false or misleading representation concerning the need for any goods or services.

Other provisions state that a person shall not, in trade or commerce, engage in conduct that is liable to mislead the public as to the nature of the manufacturing process, the characteristics, the suitability for their purpose or the quantity of any goods or services.

The ACL provides guidance as to what claims can be made about the origin of substances such as homoeopathic medicines, herbal substances and essential oils marketed as 'made in Australia' or 'product of Australia' when components of the product are from overseas. It is a matter of determining whether any claims made breach the ACL provisions that protect against false or misleading statements. Details of obligations in this area are found at: https://www.accc.gov.au/business/advertising-promoting-your-business/country-of-origin-claims.

In New South Wales, section 99 of the *Public Health Act 2010* penalises the promotion or advertisement of health services (this includes complementary medicine) that is false, misleading or deceptive, or likely to be misleading or deceptive. In addition, this provision penalises promotion or advertisement of health services that creates an unjustified expectation of beneficial treatment.

BOX 6.9

Practice tip

All these provisions raise issues for practitioners. The types of claims that might be considered to breach these provisions are:

- miracle cures of ailments
- guarantees of cures
- wonder slimming herbs or techniques
- misrepresentation of the nature of the ingredients or properties of goods or services
- misrepresentation of approval or sponsorship of goods or services (e.g. 'government approved')
- misrepresentation of the level of training or experience of the practitioner
- misrepresentation of the professional status of a practitioner (e.g. 'registered'), and
- misrepresentation of the origin of substances (e.g. 'Australian made').

National Law provisions concerning advertising (Registered Health Practitioners)

Section 133 of the National Law provides that a person should not advertise a regulated health service that is a service usually provided by a registered health practitioner—for example, a chiropractor, osteopath or Chinese medicine practitioner—in a manner that:

- is false or misleading
- offers a gift discount or other inducement unless the advertisement states the terms and conditions
- uses testimonials
- creates an unreasonable expectation of beneficial treatment, or
- directly or indirectly encourages the indiscriminate or unnecessary use of regulated health services.

There are penalties associated to breach of this provision.

Unfair contracts

The ACL may impact upon the contracts (whether oral or written) entered into by complementary medicine practitioners with consumers in some situations.

The ACL regulates unfair contract terms that are found in consumer contracts. 'Consumer contract' is defined to include a contract in standard form for a supply of goods or services to an individual whose acquisition of the goods, services or interest is wholly or predominantly for personal, domestic or household use or consumption. A term of a consumer contract is void if the term is unfair and the contract is a standard form contract.

The phrase 'standard form' is not defined, but it typically would be a contract that is brought into existence without negotiation, which involves unequal bargaining power between the parties and where there was no effective opportunity to negotiate the terms of the contract. The ACL provides that a contract is a standard form contract unless proven otherwise. An example of this type of contract is likely to be a contract that is offered on a 'take it or leave it' basis. This could occur when a complementary medicine practitioner offers orally or in writing to provide services and specifies the cost of a program of treatment and there is no negotiation as to the terms of that agreement.

This potentially would cover many transactions undertaken by complementary medicine practitioners, including sales of substances and the provision of services. The unfair contract provisions do not regulate matters such as the main subject-matter of the contract—that is, how the main subject-matter of the contract is defined, which might include the nature of the services provided. It also does not impact upon the up-front price payable under the contract, as this is a matter easily understood by consumers.

A consumer contract (or terms in that contract) may be unfair if:

* it would cause a significant imbalance in the parties' rights and obligations arising under the contract
* it is not reasonably necessary to protect the legitimate interests of the party who would be advantaged by the term, and
* it would cause detriment (whether financial or otherwise) to a party if it were to be applied or relied on.

Some examples of unfair standard forms are terms that permit one party to avoid or limit performance of the contract or permit only one party to terminate but not the other, or allow the up-front price to be varied without the right of another party to terminate the contract.

These provisions suggest that when offering to provide professional services it is important to ensure that a client is well informed about what is being offered. Any contract entered into should not rely upon the practitioner applying an unequal bargaining position against the other party; otherwise this aspect of the contract may not be enforceable.

Significant relevant case law regarding misleading and deceptive behaviour

There are a number of cases that confirm the potential liability of companies and practitioners in relation to breaches of consumer legislation. Although these cases relate to legislation in place before the commencement of the ACL, it still provides guidance as to how these types of matters may be dealt with.

In *Commissioner for Fair Trading, Department of Commerce v Hunter*,[18] an injunction was sought against a person who practised as a naturopath and medical herbalist. The primary focus of the case was in relation to his advertising of 'live blood analysis', which was said to allow diagnosis of ailments instantly and to assist in the treatment of such illnesses. The Commissioner suggested this was a misleading representation under the terms of the *Fair Trading Act 1987* (NSW). Also of concern were the representations made about the qualifications of Mr Hunter and his ability to diagnose and treat serious health conditions.

A significant issue was the fact that Mr Hunter used the titles 'Dr', 'Doctor of Natural Medicine' and 'PhD' in advertisements, together with words that could suggest he was a medical doctor. As Mr Hunter was not a medical doctor, these representations were held by the court to be misleading and deceptive representations. Also deemed to be misleading and deceptive was the representation that he was competent to treat serious illnesses such as high blood pressure and a list of other conditions. Evidence was adduced from a haematologist about the efficacy of live blood analysis and the difficulty of ascertaining medical conditions or making therapeutic decisions or diagnosis from that type of study. The court found the representations in regard to the value of live blood analysis were misleading or deceptive, or likely to mislead or deceive. The result in this case was that the court ordered that Mr Hunter be permanently restrained from carrying on a business or in any way providing in trade and commerce naturopathy, medical herbalism, herbalism, iridology, hydrotherapy, sports medicine, osteopathy and blood analysis.

Similar issues arose in the authority *Commissioner for Fair Trading, Department of Commerce v Perrett*,[19] where the Commissioner sought a declaration that the defendant had engaged in misleading or deceptive conduct and conduct likely to mislead or deceive in contravention of the *Fair Trading Act 1987* (NSW). It was also suggested he had engaged in conduct that was liable to mislead the public as to the nature, characteristics and suitability for their purpose of certain goods in contravention of section 49 of the same legislation. The Commissioner sought a restraining order in relation to these types of activities.

The case discussed the defendant's actions in relation to a number of clients involving the use of unorthodox substances of uncertain or unknown composition, the diagnosis and treatment of acute and chronic medical conditions, and the application of ointments and intravenous injections. The Commissioner suggested the defendant had represented that he had the ability to treat multiple sclerosis, breast cancer, a thyroid condition, terminal cancer, Huntington's Disease and sympathetic nerve dystrophy. The Commissioner also suggested that the defendant made statements suggesting clients should not rely upon medical treatment, and indicated he had access to knowledge and substances not normally available. The defendant was not able to present evidence to support the representations that he made about his ability to treat those ailments. On that basis, he was held to have made representations that were misleading or deceptive, or likely to mislead or deceive, and restraining orders were granted to stop that behaviour.

A significant authority dealing with misleading and deceptive behaviour relevant to complementary medicine is *Australian Competition and Consumer Commission v Purple Harmony Plates Pty Ltd*.[20] This matter related to the representations made in relation to a product called 'Purple Harmony plates', which came in different forms including disks, angels, phone disks and fridge fresheners. These products were said to have many and varied therapeutic benefits including negating the effects of electromagnetic radiation, accelerating healing, calming people, increasing health, decreasing stress levels, strengthening the immune system, and treating cuts, burns, aches and pains.

The Australian Competition and Consumer Commission (ACCC) argued that these representations, made on a website and in certain publications, suggested these products had performance characteristics they did not possess, and were misleading or deceptive or likely to mislead or deceive contrary to sections 52 and 53(c) of the *Trade Practices Act 1974* (Cth). The ACCC relied upon section 51A of the *Trade Practices Act 1974* on the basis that the representations related to future matters that could not be substantiated. This provision places the burden of proof upon a corporation that has made a representation about a future matter to demonstrate that it had reasonable grounds for making the representation; otherwise the representations will be deemed to be misleading.

The court held that the defendant had represented that the products possessed the performance characteristics claimed, and that these representations made claims as to future matters and suggested that a person who purchased the product would derive the stated benefits from the product. The defendant did not provide any substantial evidence to support the assertions made, which would address the question of whether the company had any reasonable grounds for making the representations. Accordingly, the representations were deemed to be misleading. The court ordered injunctions against making these representations and required refunds to customers and corrective advertisement.

The authority *ACCC v Nuera Health Pty Ltd. (In Liquidation)*[21] related to representations that Nuera products could cure, reverse, stop or slow the progress of cancer or prolong the life of a person suffering from cancer. The ACCC indicated that these representations suggested these products were supported by scientific evidence. Representations were made at promotional seminars and included testimonials from satisfied customers. A DVD and a website provided further representations. Nuera made statements relating to 'The Rana System', which involved treatment and diagnosis of various terminal illnesses and provided services such as fruit and vegetable diets, ozone therapy, colloidal minerals, organic oat milk and live blood viewing. Some of these treatments cost up to $35,000. Nuera did not adduce any evidence to support the claims made about its treatments. The court considered that the representations were a cynical attempt to exploit cancer victims and the representations relied upon discredited or unproven theories. The court ordered restraints on the respondents in making these representations.

The *Australian Competition and Consumer Commission v Homeopathy Plus! Australia Pty Ltd.* case[22] involved a company which sold homoeopathic products through its website and published three articles that suggested the use of homoeopathic treatment was effective and safe to deal with whooping cough and suggested the whooping cough vaccine was short lived and unreliable. The ACCC brought action suggesting this was false, misleading and/or deceptive representations contrary to ss 18 and 29 of the *Australian Consumer Law* (ACL). The respondent suggested the articles were only for general information and had a basis in homoeopathic science. This view was not accepted by Justice Perry, who considered the respondent engaged in conduct that was misleading and deceptive or likely to be so. Justice Perry considered there was no accepted evidence nor support from key homoeopathic associations for the respondent's comments.

Social media

In recent years the expansion of the use of social media such as Facebook, Twitter and Instagram has greatly increased the potential for exposure of professional health practitioners. The Australian Health Practitioner Regulation Agency's (AHPRA) National Board Policy for Registered Health Practitioners: Social Media Policy makes it clear that when using social media, health practitioners (whether registered or not) should remember their professional obligations still apply. Registered health practitioners (and in fact any health practitioner) should only post information on social media that is not in breach of professional obligations including those in regard to confidentiality, privacy or unsubstantiated claims. An example of this is the Osteopathy Board Guidelines: https://www.osteopathyboard.gov.au/Codes-Guidelines/Social-media-guidance.aspx

Liability for faulty products

A practitioner may be subject to liability where injury is caused to a client by:

*   faulty products used during treatment (e.g. contaminated massage oil)
*   adulterated herbs
*   products sold unopened that have been negligently manufactured
*   instruments with a design fault (e.g. faulty acupuncture needle causing injury to a patient), and
*   products sold with insufficient safety instructions or warnings.

Common law position

The seminal case of *Donoghue v Stevenson*,[23] which provided the modern impetus to the law relating to negligence, specifically deals with the tortious liability of a manufacturer. This case confirms that a manufacturer is liable in negligence to a person who suffers damage (including economic loss) for the shortcomings of the product. Importantly, this liability will accrue without the necessity for any contract between the manufacturer and the party injured.

The concept of a 'manufacturer' is broadly defined to include all parties in the production line, such as the manufacturer, distributor, supplier and ultimate vendor. This means that a practitioner could be deemed a manufacturer on the basis that they prepared mixtures, solutions and substances from materials purchased from other parties or that they have marketed or supplied goods to a client. This liability may apply even if they have played no role in the manufacturing of the final product.

BOX 6.10

Action plan

*   Make sure of the integrity of the manufacturers or suppliers from which you purchase your products because their negligence may affect your practice.
*   Make sure that, as far as possible, you inspect and satisfy yourself with regard to the quality and safety of goods before sale to a client.
*   Inspect machinery or instruments before use to ensure the safety of clients, staff and you.
*   Make sure that your stock is properly stored and regularly reviewed to avoid spoilage or deterioration in quality.
*   Make sure that any product sold by you displays the appropriate warnings and that clients understand its proper use and application.

The liability of a manufacturer is based on:

- whether the product was in its current form on manufacture or whether incorrect handling or storage created the dangerous condition
- whether there was an opportunity for intermediate inspection of the substance before use, which may avoid liability for the manufacturer
- whether, in the marketing of a substance or equipment, there were sufficient warnings as to correct use (some equipment is dangerous, but not if it is properly used), and
- whether the user has contributed to the injury by inappropriate action or negligent use.

Case studies

Sealed container of adulterated health product

A naturopath purchases a sealed container containing a natural health product from a major manufacturer. He sells the unopened product to a client as treatment. If the product—normally harmless—is adulterated with a harmful ingredient, the manufacturer would *prima facie* be liable for the injury or economic loss suffered by the client. Any liability in negligence for the naturopath would probably be avoided, assuming that the substance was not harmful in its non-adulterated form and that the practitioner has not done anything to the substance or allowed the substance to deteriorate by inappropriate storage. Liability for the sale of goods that are not merchantable or not in accordance with description may still apply against the practitioner under the SGA, as there is strict liability under these provisions. The practitioner could most likely join the manufacturer in any action taken against them under the SGA, or seek contribution for any liability he or she may have.

Adulterated herbs

A herbalist purchases raw herbs from a wholesaler. The herbs are adulterated and a client is poisoned. If the contamination was not detectable and there was no reason to suspect that the herbs were contaminated, the practitioner may not be liable as a manufacturer. There may be liability against the practitioner for a breach of the condition of merchantability, or for not being in conformity with description pursuant to the SGA. The manufacturer would be liable to the consumer for the breach of the obligation to use reasonable care in manufacturing or processing.

Acupuncture needle breaks

An acupuncturist uses an acupuncture needle that breaks on entry into the body because the needle was not properly manufactured. Surgical removal is required. Assuming that it can be shown that the needle was negligently manufactured, unless the manufacturer can show there was inappropriate use of the needle by the practitioner or unusual force used, the manufacturer will be liable directly to the client.

Homoeopathic substance poisons

If homoeopathic substances are distilled by a homoeopath into a tincture, the homoeopath is in that case a manufacturer in relation to that combination. The manufacturer of the mother tincture provides materials that may be poisonous by themselves with the intention that the homoeopath should produce a dilution to safe levels. If by error the homoeopath produced a tincture where the concentration was at poisonous levels, the homoeopath would be liable in negligence for any injury to a client under the common law relevant to manufacturers and under the SGA conditions. No liability would accrue to the manufacturer of the mother tincture unless there was unclear or incorrect labelling. If the mother tincture was incorrectly labelled as to the substances contained in the tincture or as to its concentration, it is likely that any injury would be the responsibility of the manufacturer of that tincture. A practitioner's potential liability as a manufacturer or under the SGA confirms the necessity to secure reliable sources for herbs, vitamins and therapeutic substances.

The Australian Consumer Law Parts 3–5

The ACL[24] contains provisions that allow an action against a manufacturer of goods if the goods have a safety defect that has caused injury. These provisions provide a statutory liability not based on contract or tort, and may provide an easier means to enforce the manufacturer's liability.

The basic scheme of these provisions is to make a corporation liable for the manufacturing of goods in trade or commerce that have a defect. Goods are deemed to 'have a defect if their safety is not such as persons generally are entitled to expect'.[25] 'Manufacturer' is defined to include a person who 'grows, extracts, produces, processes or assembles goods'.[26]

Notes

1 *Therapeutic Goods (Victoria) Act 2010* (Vic); *Poisons and Therapeutic Goods Act 1966* (NSW); *Therapeutic Goods Act 2001* (Tas); *Controlled Substances Act 1984* (SA) s 11 A; *Therapeutic Goods Act 2019* (Qld).
2 Commonwealth Constitution, s 51(i), (xx), (xxiiiA).
3 Bensoussan & Myers, *Towards a Safer Choice*, p. 234.
4 TGA, Australian regulatory guidelines for complementary medicines (ARGCM) version 1.0 May 2020 p. 9. https://www.tga.gov.au/publication/australian-regulatory-guidelines-listed-medicines-and-registered-complementary-medicines (accessed 2 November 2021).
5 *Therapeutic Goods Act* (Cmth) ss 14 and 14 A.
6 Bensoussan & Myers, *Towards a Safer Choice*, p. 236.
7 *Therapeutic Goods Act* (Cth) s 31.
8 https://www.tga.gov.au/sites/default/files/general_guidance_for_listed_medicines_formerly_argcm_part_b.pdf page 4 (accessed 2 November 2021).
9 https://www.tga.gov.au/assessed-listed-medicines (accessed 2 November 2021).
10 https://www.tga.gov.au/publication/australian-regulatory-guidelines-listed-medicines-and-registered-complementary-medicines (accessed 2 November 2021).
11 Defined in Regulation 2 as 'a preparation a. formulated for use on the principle that it is capable of producing in a healthy person symptoms similar to those which it is administered to alleviate; and b. prepared according to the practices of homoeopathic pharmacy using the methods of: i. Serial dilution and succussion of a mother tincture in water, ethanol, aqueous ethanol or glycerol; or ii. Serial trituration in lactose'.

12 https://www.legislation.gov.au/Series/F2016L01287 (accessed 2 November 2021).
13 www.medsafe.govt.nz/profs/NaturalHealth.asp (accessed 15 July 2021).
14 https://www.accc.gov.au/publications/advertising-selling (accessed 20 October 2021).
15 'Goods' is defined as 'all chattels personal other than things in action and money, and also includes emblements and things attached to or forming part of the land which are agreed to be severed before sale or under the contract of sale'.
16 Australian Consumer Law (ACL), ss 54–56.
17 Australian Consumer Law, Section 4B.
18 [2008] NSWSC 277.
19 [2007] NSWSC 1130 (12 October 2007).
20 [2001] FCA 1062 (6 August 2001).
21 [2007] FCA 695 (9 May 2007).
22 (2014) 146 ALD 278; [2014] FCA 1412.
23 [1932] AC 562.
24 *Australian Consumer Law*, ss 138–142.
25 *Australian Consumer Law*, s 9.
26 *Australian Consumer Law*, s 7.

Resources

T. Addison, *Negligent Failure to Inform* (2003) 11 *Torts Law Journal* 165.

Australian Competition and Consumer Commission: www.accc.gov.au (health services and relevant trade practices issues).

Australian Health Practitioner Regulation Agency: www.ahpra.gov.au/Notifications.aspx.

B. Bennett & I. Freckelton, 'Life After the IPP Reforms: Medical Negligence Law', in I. Freckelton & K. Petersen (eds), *Disputes and Dilemmas in Health Law*, Federation Press, Sydney, 2006.

R.J. Douglas, G.R. Mullins & S.R. Grant, *The Annotated Civil Liability Act 2003 (Qld)*, 3rd ed., Lexis Nexis Butterworths, Sydney, 2012.

S. Todd (ed.), *The Law of Torts in New Zealand*, 4th ed., Thomson Brookers, Wellington, 2005.

P. Vines, 'Apologizing to Avoid Liability: Cynical Civility or Practical Morality' (2005) *Sydney Law Review* 483.

M. Weir, 'Obligation to Advise of Options of Treatment—Medical Doctors and Complementary and Alternative Medicine Practitioners' (2003) 10 *Journal of Law and Medicine* 296–307.

In addition, the Therapeutic Goods Administration at www.tga.gov.au offers a number of extremely useful resources, such as: 'An Overview of the Regulation of Complementary Medicines in Australia', www.tga.gov.au/overview-regulation-complementary-medicines-australia, and the Australian Regulatory Guidelines for Complementary Medicines (ARGCM), www.tga.gov.au/publication/australian-regulatory-guidelines-complementary-medicines-argcm.

7   Modalities

This chapter raises some of the most important issues applicable to specific modalities. Although all practitioners need to be concerned with ethical and legal considerations, some issues are modality specific or loom larger for particular modalities. For example, the skin-penetration provisions are especially important for acupuncturists; the *Therapeutic Goods Act* is particularly relevant for homoeopaths, TCM practitioners or herbalists; and the risk of neck manipulation is particularly important for chiropractors and osteopaths. This chapter highlights some significant Australian Health Practitioners Regulation Agency (AHPRA) Codes and Guidelines for registered practitioners. Reference to specific modality Codes and Guidelines for a registered practitioner is necessary.

AHPRA Codes and Guidelines

AHPRA provides a number of Codes and Guidelines that are applicable for all registered health practitioners including complementary medicine practitioners. The Codes and Guidelines include:

Advertising for Registered Practitioners

In December 2020 the 'Guidelines for Advertising as Regulated Health Services' was released outlining the obligations for registered practitioners.[1] Further details and information for practitioners, advertisers, consumers and the public is provided in the Advertising Hub including information about making a complaint and frequently asked questions.[2] Understanding the obligations of a practitioner in relation to advertising is important as AHPRA has been active in enforcing these advertising guidelines and in some cases it has brought legal actions against practitioners if a breach occurs.

There are resources to assist in the application of the advertising guidelines covering:

- Acceptable evidence in health advertising
- Summary of the advertising requirements
- Common examples of non-compliant advertising
- Self-assessment tool
- Testimonials: Understand the requirements
- Using titles in health advertising tool
- Chinese medicine examples of non-compliant advertising
- Position statement on Chinese medicine practitioners making therapeutic claims in advertising

DOI: 10.4324/9781003195931-7

Code of Conduct

Twelve National Boards have developed a generic Code of Conduct that focusses on:[3]

1 Put patients first – Safe, effective and collaborative Practice
    1.1   Providing good care
    1.2   Good care
    1.3   Decisions about access to car
    1.4   Treatment in emergencies
2 Aboriginal and Torres Strait Islander health and cultural Safety
    2.1   Aboriginal and/or Torres Strait Islander health
    2.2   Cultural safety for Aboriginal and Torres Strait Islander Peoples
3 Respectful and culturally safe practice for all
    3.1   Cultural safety for all communities
    3.2   Effective communication
    3.3   Confidentiality and privacy
    3.4   End-of-life care
4 Working with patients
    4.1   Partnership
    4.2   Informed consent
    4.3   Children, young people and other patients who may have additional needs
    4.4   Relatives, carers and partners
    4.5   Adverse events and open disclosure
    4.6   Complaints
    4.7   Ending a professional relationship
    4.8   Personal relationships
    4.9   Professional boundaries
    4.10 Working with multiple patients
    4.11 Closing or relocating a practice
5 Working with other practitioners
    5.1   Respect for colleagues and other practitioners
    5.2   Teamwork and collaboration
    5.3   Discrimination, bullying and harassment
    5.4   Delegation, referral and handover
6 Working within the healthcare system
    6.1   Use healthcare resources wisely
    6.2   Health advocacy
    6.3   Public health
7 Minimising risk to patients
    7.1   Risk management
    7.2   Practitioner performance
    7.3   Maintaining and developing professional capability
    7.4   Continuing professional development (CPD).

The AHPRA provides Guidelines about significant issues for practitioners. See notes 4 and 5 below: 'Social Media—How to meet your obligations under the National Law'[4] and 'Mandatory notifications about registered health practitioners'.[5]

BOX 7.1

Action plan

- Base diagnosis and clinical practice on good-quality x-ray evidence.
- Refer clients to medical doctors when a medical problem is evident.
- Test for any contraindications to treatment.
- Do not use the term 'doctor' without qualifiers, to avoid holding out as a medical doctor.

Chiropractic

The major concerns for chiropractors are the role of diagnosis, the appropriate use of x-rays, the clinical consequences of cervical spine manipulation and the use of the term 'doctor'.

The role of a chiropractor

The role of a medical practitioner involves the diagnosis of disease states based on symptoms, medical tests and assessments. Historically, chiropractors have avoided the use of the term 'diagnosis', preferring terms such as 'analysis' or 'assessment'. This approach was partially motivated by a desire to avoid the implication that chiropractors were engaged in the practice of medicine at a time when this was an offence in some jurisdictions in the United States. Since chiropractors long ago attained registered status, and the legislative provisions limiting 'the practice of medicine' to medical doctors have been repealed in Australia, this should no longer be a concern—though it is important for a chiropractor to practise within the accepted scope of practice for chiropractic.

A chiropractor is obliged to recognise medical conditions to ascertain whether he or she should or could treat that condition. If a client comes to a chiropractor with a known medical condition, the chiropractor needs to establish whether chiropractic can provide benefits for the client. If not, the practitioner should explain this to the client and consider whether a referral to a medical practitioner or other health professional is required. If treatment of the client is undertaken, the limits of chiropractic treatment should be explained and the client encouraged not to abandon medical options.

Use of x-ray evidence

Interpretation of x-rays

At the core of chiropractic practice is the identification of chiropractic subluxations, sometimes using x-rays. This technique brings with it the need for responsible and competent use of the information obtained. Is a chiropractor liable in negligence for the interpretation of the results of an x-ray? If a chiropractor doesn't perceive a fracture shown on an x-ray, does that create liability for any resulting injury?

The chiropractor's actions will be assessed against the standard of competent practice based on peer professional opinion in accordance with the standard set by the civil liability legislation. If a chiropractor acting in accordance with that standard would not have seen the fracture, then this would support an argument that no negligence has occurred. If the fracture was not seen because the x-ray was of poor quality, a court may conclude that another x-ray should have been taken. It has been said that a poor x-ray is as bad as no x-ray.

Adjustments resulting in injury and made without a satisfactory x-ray may be negligent if expert evidence indicates that an x-ray should have been taken and would have revealed the potential for injury.

Interpretation of medical conditions

More problematic is the issue of whether chiropractors are liable for not noticing a condition such as a cancerous growth or pneumonia revealed by an x-ray. Arguably, those types of conditions are not within the scope of a chiropractor's practice, which is centred on the neuromusculoskeletal system.

If competent professional practice based on peer professional opinion suggests that the chiropractor should have understood the nature of the condition revealed by the x-ray, this could provide the grounds for liability. In one US authority, a chiropractor was deemed negligent in not detecting a cancer on an x-ray taken for the purpose of chiropractic adjustments. The court accepted evidence from a medical doctor that the chiropractor should have been able to identify the abnormality and then refer to a medical practitioner who could make that diagnosis.[6] If practitioners are concerned about the quality of x-rays, it may be advisable to refer to a radiologist. The Chiropractic Board of Australia in the Guideline in relation to Radiology/Radiography provides guidance in relation to the appropriate use of these facilities:

> Chiropractors must comply with the provisions of the code of practice for radiation protection and the RPS 19 *Code of Practice for Radiation Protection in the Application of Ionizing Radiation Chiropractors* (2009) or any subsequent version as published by the Australian Radiation Protection and Nuclear Safety Agency (ARPANSA Code), and applicable Commonwealth, state or territory laws in relation to best practice.
>
> (www.chiropracticboard.gov.au/Codes-guidelines/FAQ/
> Conduct-performance/Chiropractic-diagnostic-imaging.aspx)

Adverse reactions

Risks of cervical spine manipulation

Although chiropractic has an impressive safety record, there is a perception by some that one risk of chiropractic is the possibility of stroke caused by cervical spine manipulation.[7] On many occasions, what is portrayed as a stroke or cerebrovascular injury caused by chiropractic manipulation is in fact the result of manipulation by a medical practitioner, untrained manipulator or family member.[8] Despite this apparent distortion, there is evidence that on very rare occasions chiropractic cervical spine manipulation may cause strokes and other less serious results.[9]

The calculation of the risk of complication caused by cervical spine manipulation varies widely, depending on the seriousness of the reactions. Less serious reactions such as post-manipulative diffuse pain lasting less than two days have been quoted as occurring in 40 per cent of cases, and fainting, cold perspiration and nausea as occurring in one to two cases out of 1,000.[10] In relation to manipulations causing death, figures are quoted suggesting that this event occurs in one out of ten million manipulations or tens of millions of manipulations, while serious reactions occur in one in one million adjustments or one in 400,000 adjustments.[11]

The causes of the more serious incidents could be the result of factors such as:[12]

- inadequate diagnostic habits
- inadequate x-ray evaluation
- delay in referral
- delay in re-evaluation
- lack of inter-professional cooperation
- ignoring patient intolerances
- poor technique selection, and
- poor technique.

Precautions

Because of the potential for serious complications from manipulation, practitioners should consider clinical precautions such as diagnostic tests to ascertain high-risk clients. For clients considered high risk, the chiropractor could decline treatment, vary the type of manipulation provided and/or refer to a medical practitioner. Contraindications to manipulation may include arthritis, recent trauma such as whiplash, osteoporosis, circulatory disturbances, neurological dysfunction or vertigo. If injury is caused to a client where clear contraindications existed, that may provide grounds for a claim in negligence.

The civil liability legislation in New South Wales, Queensland, Victoria, South Australia and Western Australia provides that a person is not liable for the materialisation of an inherent risk, which is a risk of something occurring that cannot be avoided by the exercise of reasonable care and skill. This may assist a chiropractor in resisting a negligence claim for an adverse result. These provisions do not affect the obligation to warn of risks of treatment.

Duty to advise of the risks of stroke or other reactions

The authority of *Rogers v Whitaker* (pages 122–123) provides a fairly strict test of the risks for which a warning should be given by a medical practitioner. In that case, a complication said to occur in one out of 14,000 operations required a risk warning.

The decision to advise of a risk depends on the seriousness of the potential injury, the nature of the procedure, the desire of the client for information, the temperament and health of the client, and the general surrounding circumstances. Even if the practitioner is not negligent in the chiropractic treatment provided, liability may arise where a client is not properly advised of the risks of treatment. For example, if a client suffers a rare but not unforeseeable reaction and faints, causing physical injury, the lack of warning may be negligent even if the treatment was competently performed.

The practice of the profession does not determine a practitioner's obligation to warn of risks. This is a matter for the courts. Authorities suggest that, even if the complication is rare, the client should be warned—especially when it may have an impact on the client's decision to undertake the treatment.

It would be good professional practice to advise of common minor reactions to manipulation, such as perspiration or diffuse pain. Fainting is not a common reaction, but the possible consequences of this complication are serious. It is recommended that warning of this reaction should be given before treatment. Procedures should be put into place to ensure that clients do not leave supervision until the initial reactions to manipulation may have subsided.

In relation to possible death or strokes, the question is more difficult. A warning of this improbable complication will protect against negligence for insufficient warnings of risks of treatment. It is appreciated that this may be a confronting activity for a practitioner but the potentially catastrophic impact of that consequence of treatment would suggest the need to warn.

If a practitioner chooses not to warn of the risk of death, stroke or other serious reaction, a claim made that insufficient warnings of risk were given might be met by the following arguments:

*   Any level of risk discussed by the literature suggests that this complication is *extremely* rare and, in considering the factors discussed in *Rogers v Whitaker*, there was no legal requirement to warn of that risk.
*   The practitioner took steps to vary manipulations to take this risk into account.
*   It is not the profession's practice to warn of this risk (this is not determinative).
*   Even if warned of the risk, the client would have continued with the procedure— that is, causation is absent.

Use of the title 'doctor'

Some chiropractors use the titles 'doctor or 'Dr', either with or without the letters DC or the words 'chiropractor' or 'chiropractic'. Section 4.4.3 of the AHPRA Guidelines for Advertising a Regulated Health Services indicates that there is no provision in the National Law specifically prohibiting a chiropractor from using titles such as 'doctor' but there is potential for the use of this title to mislead or deceive.

Reference is made to sections 116 and 117 of the National Law, which prohibit a practitioner or person from knowingly or recklessly taking or using any title that could be reasonably understood to induce a belief that the practitioner is registered in a health profession or a division of a health profession in which the practitioner or person is not registered. This should always be borne in mind when using terms like 'Dr'.

The guidelines do indicate that if the title 'Dr' is used in advertising, and the practitioner is not a registered medical practitioner, then it should be made clear that the practitioner does not hold registration as a medical practitioner—for example, by including a reference to their health profession whenever the title is used, such as Dr Mary Jones (Chiropractor). In any event, the type of advertising used should not represent the practitioner as having qualifications, endorsement or registration that they do not possess.

Pre-paid treatment plans

Some chiropractors provide clients with the option of entering into a treatment plan that involves pre-payment for treatment over a period of time. This has been a matter of some concern over a number of years, owing to the perception by some that this may entrench over-servicing without proper clinical justification, to the detriment of the client. Clause 4.2 (e) of the AHPRA Code of Conduct provides some general guidance on this issue.

This issue was reflected in clause 3.6 of the Code of Conduct for Chiropractors produced by the Chiropractic Board of Australia (now superseded). Although the terms of clause 3.6 do not appear under the new AHPRA Code of Conduct commenced in 2022 the comments below are good practice and new guidelines may be provided later. The superseded Code of Conduct required chiropractors to consider the following when finalising these agreements:

- The practitioner should ensure that the client clearly understands the nature of all of the terms and conditions of the agreement, which have been fully disclosed.
- The plan should be based upon the clinical needs of the patient.
- The agreement should incorporate a reasonable 'cooling-off' period, allowing the client to decide not to continue with an agreement after signature.
- The client should also be offered a 'pay-as-you-go' option.
- The agreement should include provision for a reasonable refund for any unused period of treatment after early termination.
- There should be no financial disadvantage for the early termination of the agreement based upon Australian Consumer Law requirements discussed above at pages 158–159.
- There should be no difference in the quality of care provided to those on a pre-paid treatment plan and those who are not.
- The agreement should be reviewed every three months or every twelve visits, whichever is the longer period.
- The agreement should not extend beyond three months or twelve visits, whichever is the longer period, unless there is clear clinical justification for a renewal.[13]

The provisions of the Australian Consumer Law that will apply across Australia (discussed on pages 156–161) suggest the need for great care to ensure that these contracts are properly negotiated and do not contain provisions that might be considered unfair based upon a use of unequal bargaining power between the practitioner and the client.

Patient records

Chiropractors and other health professionals need to consider clause 8.3 of the AHPRA Code of Conduct which deals with the obligations to provide good quality patient records.[14] dealing with obligations to complete and keep professional records that should be understood, as they may be referred to in any proceedings brought against a practitioner by a client, AHPRA, the Chiropractic Board of Australia or other body.

Position statement—March 2019 interim policy on spinal
manipulation for infants and young children

The interim policy suggests 'chiropractors to not use spinal manipulation to treat children under two years of age, pending the recommendations arising from the independent expert review' subject to a review by Safer Care Victoria.[15] Refer to note 16 below.[16]

Advertising

In addition to the generic AHPRA guidelines for advertising above there are specific chiropractic information below about Chiropractic examples of non-compliant advertising.[17]

Examples of chiropractic misconduct for consideration

Chiropractic is overall a very safe modality but on occasions chiropractors may be found to have been involved in misconduct. The following examples may provide some insight into what actions should be avoided.

- A chiropractor was found guilty of professional misconduct by the Health Care Complaints Commission and was given a 2 year cancellation and a prohibition order for posting articles that suggested chiropractic could treat or cure cancer. This was seen to be unethical, unprofessional and a patent disregard of professional standards.
- A chiropractor was disqualified permanently because of a tendency to subject female patients to inappropriate physical contact.[18]
- A chiropractor was found not to have held professional indemnity insurance for about 16 months and provided a false declaration to AHPRA. The chiropractor was subject to a condition to provide evidence of insurance on an ongoing basis.[19]
- A person who purported to be a registered chiropractor, medical practitioner and acupuncturist and was holding out as a registered health practitioner was found guilty of holding out in breach of sections 113 and 116 of the *Health Practitioner Regulation National Law.*[20]

Osteopathy

This modality is a 'whole-body' system of manual therapy, based on unique bio-mechanical principles, which uses a wide range of techniques to treat musculoskeletal problems and other functional disorders of the body.

Osteopaths are primary care practitioners, and are trained to recognise conditions that require medical referral. They are also trained to carry out standard medical examinations of the cardiovascular, respiratory and nervous systems.

Chiropractic emphasises manipulations of the spine and its articulations. Osteopaths concern themselves less with spinal manipulation and more with techniques associated with functional therapies, muscle energy techniques and techniques designed to deal with malfunctions of the internal organs and bio-mechanics. Unlike chiropractors, osteopaths rarely use x-rays as a diagnostic technique. Osteopathy has a close association with orthodox medicine, based on its concern with a broad range of therapies directed to treatment of the blood supply, lymphatic drainage and skeletal disorders.

BOX 7.2

Action plan

Make sure you follow the Osteopathy Board of Australia's Guidelines for Advertising a Regulated Health Service (s 4.1.4) on the use of the term 'Dr' or 'doctor'.

The role of an osteopath

An osteopath is obliged to recognise medical conditions to ascertain whether he or she should or could treat that condition. If the client comes to an osteopath with a known medical condition, it is the responsibility of the osteopath to determine whether osteopathy can provide benefits for the client. If not, the practitioner should explain this to the client and should consider referral to a medical practitioner or other health professional. If treatment of the client is undertaken, the limits of osteopathy treatment should be explained and the client encouraged not to abandon medical options.

Use of the term 'doctor'

See the discussion on this point relating to chiropractors on page 171. Similar considerations apply to osteopaths.

Patient records

Osteopaths and other health professional need to consider clause 8.3 of the AHPRA Code of Conduct that deals with obligations to keep complete professional records. This needs to be understood as they may be referred to in any proceedings brought against a practitioner https://www.ahpra.gov.au/Publications/Code-of-conduct.aspx.

Therapeutic massage and myotherapy

The general term 'therapeutic massage' includes a large number of massage modalities, such as sports massage, shiatsu, kahuna massage, Swedish massage and deep-tissue massage. Each modality has its own approach and philosophy, but generally involves a system of manual application of massage by the hand, foot, knee and elbow to superficial tissue by the use of techniques including stroking, kneading, cupping and vibration. This section will discuss issues relevant to all these modalities generally, with reference to particular modalities where necessary. Therapeutic massage usually involves the use of massage oil, often in conjunction with aromatherapy treatment.

BOX 7.3

Action plan

- Don't diagnose.
- Don't manipulate the cervical spine.

- Don't massage where it may cause or aggravate injury or cause adverse skin reactions.
- Be sensitive to client privacy and the need for careful practices with regard to disrobing.
- Take great care in advertising to attract genuine clientele.
- Take precautions to protect your personal safety.

Restricted acts

The significant issue for massage therapists can be found in section 123 of the National Law, which limits 'manipulation of the cervical spine' to medical doctors, chiropractors, osteopaths and physiotherapists. This is defined as 'moving the joints of the cervical spine beyond a person's usual physiological range of motion using a high velocity, low amplitude thrust'. Refer to the discussion in the next section in relation to ensuring that your practice as a massage therapist does not breach this provision. Similar considerations apply in New Zealand.

A massage therapist should never manipulate the cervical spine. It doesn't matter whether the client suffers injury by that manipulation or not—the offence will occur under the National Law. Substantial monetary penalties can apply to such an act.

On occasion, a vertebra may be adjusted as an indirect result of the relaxation and muscular release associated with a massage. This is unlikely to constitute a breach of this provision, as it is an unintended result of the massage. The same could not be said for a massage technique that has as its intention—albeit indirectly—the adjustment of the cervical spine. In the South Australian District Court case of *Edwards v Butler*,[21] a massage therapist was deemed to have breached his contractual obligations and been negligent after a finding that he had applied a manipulation to the neck of a client who suffered injury.

Scope of practice

Although the National Law does not contain broad scope of practice provisions vested only in registered health practitioners, it is good practice for massage therapists to be aware of the nature of the modality to ensure that their practice remains within the accepted boundaries of the profession.

A massage therapist should not diagnose illness or disease. This is the role of medical doctors and other professions. The training and experience of massage therapists does not equip them with the knowledge to undertake the responsibility for diagnosis. A client may rely on your 'diagnosis' and not seek the medical or other assistance that may be necessary.

For example, a client may mention they have a bad back, sore neck or skin lesion. A massage therapist should not offer opinions that the client may have a specific medical condition. A client may comment about a sore on their leg that is taking a long time to heal. You might reply that the healing is slow there because the blood supply is not good to that part of the body. This may encourage a client not to seek medical examination for what could be a skin cancer, and this may be to the detriment of the client. If a client raises a health issue, or if you are concerned about an aspect of the client's health, ask the client to seek medical advice and/or, in the case of back problems, to seek the services of a chiropractor or osteopath. A practitioner should never advise a client to stop taking prescribed medicines or discourage a client from continuing medical or other professional assistance.

Use of oils

The practice of therapeutic massage will usually involve the application of massage oil with other substances as part of an aromatherapy treatment. A client's skin may have an adverse reaction to these oils and substances, and a practitioner should take this possibility into account. Before the massage starts, the practitioner should ascertain whether the client is aware of any adverse reactions they have previously had to massage oil, herbs, fragrances or other substances. A pre-massage test on a sensitive area, either behind the ear or on the wrist, may quickly indicate whether a reaction is likely.

BOX 7.4

Practice tip

If, while massaging, there appears to be an adverse skin reaction, action should be taken to remove the oil. If a reaction happens after the massage, this should be noted on the client's record. Liability for a serious skin reaction would depend on whether the practitioner had applied oil of a type and in a manner consistent with standard professional practice. If the same client had a second reaction when the same oil was applied, it would be difficult to argue that there had not been negligence by the practitioner.

Sexual behaviour and massage

The public profile of this profession is unfortunately clouded by the perception that there is a relationship between massage therapy and the sex industry. The sex industry uses therapeutic massage to provide an acceptable public face to its industry while providing, in advertising and promotion, coded messages as to what services are available. Advertising and promotion by the sex industry will often involve reference to massage, massage parlours, relaxation centres and similar terms to indicate the availability of sexual services. As a result, professional practitioners of therapeutic massage need to consider:

- the need to differentiate their services from those of the sex industry
- potential claims for misconduct of a sexual nature that may be made against practitioners, which requires special consideration of advertising and promotion, clinic set-up and client dealings, and
- security issues.

Most massage therapy students enter professional education with strong intrinsic altruistic values to help others.[22] 'TM occupies a unique position as against other hands-on bodywork therapies'[23] that has created a difficult environment for the professionalisation of the profession. In an environment where it is easy to call oneself a massage therapist with little or no training or qualifications there is limited control over entry to the profession. This has been exacerbated by the reality of the practice of therapeutic massage. Therapeutic massage will normally involve a client in a relatively unsupervised and private place with the client alone with the practitioner. The client will normally be supine in a state of undress other than underpants.[24]

The massage will normally involve the massage of most of the body other than breast tissue and genital areas. There is nothing necessarily illegal in massaging the breast and genital areas but this is an act which would require the clear consent of the client and an information rich environment where there are acknowledged purposes and benefits for that activity. In a professional context this would not normally not arise, as codes of conduct for most therapeutic massage professional associations indicate massage of these areas is not permitted[25] or there are specific consent requirements for that practice.[26]

One aspect of good professional practice is a very careful description of what is intended to be done as part of the massage treatment, including whether buttocks are included. For some massage therapists (some of whom are either not trained at all or are trained at a low level) the combination of these circumstances has led to temptation. This have led to charges, convictions, complaints and prohibition orders dealing with sexual assault and rape during the provision of therapeutic massage. Therapeutic massage professional associations and educators have been awake to this issue and have normally applied professional level educational standards for membership and CPE training dealing with matters relevant to this issue. The control of such behaviour is currently regulated through:

- criminal law proceedings for sexual assault or rape which have deterrence impacts
- professional association discipline which may lead to expulsion though not necessarily stopping membership of another professional association
- loss of access to health fund rebates
- health complaints legislation and codes of conduct for Unregistered Health Practitioners potentially leading to an interim or permanent prohibition order in NSW, Qld, Victoria and SA.

BOX 7.5

Practice tip: Advertising

Avoid advertising in those sections of newspapers used by massage parlours and escort agencies. Even if you use terms such as 'strictly therapeutic massage only' or 'qualified massage therapist', if this advertisement is among non-genuine advertisements, it may attract those not genuinely interested in your services. The best and probably most secure means to increase your clientele is by word of mouth, by referral from other practitioners such as chiropractors or naturopaths, and by speaking to sporting clubs and community groups

Practice tip: Personal safety

It will not always be possible to be accompanied by another person for personal protection when performing massage therapy. The following are therefore useful tips:

- Screen telephone contacts by asking where they found out about your services. If the source is not a trusted friend or client, or you sense that they may be seeking services you do not offer, indicating the nature of your services may give an opportunity for a reaction.

- There are a number of signs that sexual massage is being sought. This could be when the prospective client uses terms such as 'Are there any extras?' or 'Can I get a release?' or reference to your age, looks or tipping.
- In relation to new clients, ask for first and last name with a telephone number for confirmation. A genuine caller will probably have no problem with this requirement. On confirmation, note whether there is some doubt about whether they have provided their true name.
- Avoid booking a new client as the last client of the day, as the presence of another client may be helpful should it be necessary to ask the new client to leave.
- Avoid creating an impression by your demeanour or dress that you are anything other than a professional therapeutic massage therapist.
- Your normal pre-massage interview for a new client, where you find out about their medical history and other details, should indicate clearly the nature of the services provided, the level of undressing required, draping procedures and those areas massaged and not massaged.
- Note any signs of sexual arousal. These may not indicate that a client is interested in sex but may be a normal physiological reaction. However, if the body language, words or sounds indicate that the client is interested in sex, confront the client and, if you are not satisfied with the reply, terminate the massage.
- Remember that you are in control of the provision of professional services. Your ability to convey this control in a confident and professional manner will help you avoid these circumstances and will assist in their resolution if they do occur.

The massage

Consent

A client is entitled to be given details of the types of services that are to be provided. This is part of the obligation for obtaining consent to the touching of a client. It is important for both parties to understand their expectations about the services being provided. This is a good opportunity for a client to air any concerns he or she may have. Some clients may be uncomfortable about being undressed in the presence of a stranger. It would be advisable to indicate that underclothes will remain on at all times. If massage of the buttocks is intended, this should be explained. It should be discussed whether the client's breasts will be massaged. Some professional associations have a policy that breasts should not be massaged.

You should indicate the arrangements that will be made for draping the parts of the body not being worked on. The client should be given an opportunity to ask questions or raise any objections, as they may prefer that some parts of the body not be touched.

Although it is legally possible for a person to give consent to massage in relation to intimate areas of the body in a professional context, massage of intimate areas of a client should not occur as the potential for misunderstanding is so great. Many professional associations expressly forbid that type of massage.

A Victorian case involved a claim brought against a male massage therapist after he massaged the buttocks of a female client. The client was distressed by this action and commenced an action for sexual harassment against the practitioner under the Victorian equal opportunity legislation. The massage therapist was successful in defending the action on the basis that it was not shown that there was a sexual element in his actions. It would appear that a more detailed discussion of the nature of the massage to be provided may have avoided this dispute. This discussion may have provided an opportunity for the client to indicate her requirements clearly.

Contraindications to massage

Practitioners need to understand and observe the contraindications to massage. These conditions would include cancer, heart disease, stroke, thrombosis, recent surgery, skin lesions, injury such as a fracture, suspected fracture or muscular injury where massage may cause more damage, osteoporosis or pregnancy. If faced with these conditions, a practitioner might decide not to massage, refer the client to a medical doctor or other practitioner, or vary the techniques used to avoid any injury occurring to the client. It is essential that a practitioner obtain a sufficient degree of medical information from a client to be able to determine whether any contraindications exist in relation to that client.

Naturopathy

A naturopath employs the 'nature cure', which emphasises attention to diet, exercise and fasting. Naturopathy may be employed with other modalities such as iridology, therapeutic massage, acupuncture and homoeopathic remedies. The emphasis in naturopathy is on assisting the recuperative and healing powers of the body to work effectively—that is, for the body to heal itself.

BOX 7.6

Action plan

- Test for adverse reactions to substances given to clients.
- Take care in the advocacy of diets and regimes that may cause harm to susceptible persons such as diabetics.

Adverse reactions

At-risk substances

Some substances have the potential for adverse reactions. There is evidence of some negative reactions in relation to royal jelly, echinacea and many other substances. Careful attention needs to be given to obtaining information from clients to ascertain any previous evidence of adverse reaction. It may be appropriate to suggest minimal doses at the start of treatment for substances known to cause adverse reactions, and for clients to be educated as to the signs of an adverse reaction so that treatment is ceased immediately.

Reaction to pharmaceuticals

There is a possibility of incompatibility of naturopathic regimes with pharmaceuticals prescribed by a medical doctor. Practitioners should ascertain the nature of any pharmaceuticals being used by a client and ensure that there will be no adverse reaction between these substances. Clients should not be advised to stop taking medicines prescribed by medical doctors.

Diets

An important aspect of a naturopath's practice is advice to clients on preferred diet practices. This will often be a focus of the treatment suggested. On most occasions, the diets prescribed are undoubtedly beneficial but practitioners should be aware that some clients might be susceptible to illness.

Diabetics

Diabetics may be susceptible to illness if insufficient food or the wrong type of food is eaten. The client may not be aware of this susceptibility, as many diabetics are undiagnosed. If necessary, a referral to a medical doctor to test for this condition may be prudent.

Persons with imbalances

Clients may have hormonal imbalances or be mineral depleted because of illness, prescribed drugs or pharmaceutical substances. A specific diet may accentuate this imbalance. If it could be shown that a diet suggested by a naturopath worsened, contributed to or caused this to occur, then this may result in liability for negligent advice or a failure to warn of the risks of treatment.

Radical diets

Any diets that might be perceived as radical in nature, such as fasting or water-only diets, raise particular potential liability issues for practitioners. The possible consequences of such a regime should be carefully considered and monitored by a practitioner to avoid injury to a client. The more radical the remedy suggested by the practitioner, the greater the care needed.

Homoeopathy

Homoeopathy relies on the basic principle of *similia similibus curentur* (the law of similars), which suggests that a practitioner should prescribe extremely dilute tinctures of substances that produce in healthy persons similar symptoms to the malady being treated. This is designed to stimulate the body's own healing ability.

> **BOX 7.7**
> ___
>
> **Action plan**
>
> * Make sure that all substances used comply with the *Therapeutic Goods Act* or are exempt.
> * Take care when prescribing potentially poisonous substances.
> * Levy goods and services tax on services if you are registered for this tax.

Compliance with the Therapeutic Goods Act

Refer to the discussion of the important provisions of this legislation in Chapter 6. Most practitioners will purchase homoeopathic substances in ready-made form for supply to a client. If this is intended, the provisions of the TGA exempt them if they are sufficiently dilute—that is, less than a one thousand-fold dilution.

If a practitioner intends to prepare his or her own homoeopathic substances from a mother tincture, further considerations apply. To manufacture in this way requires the substance to be registered or listed in the name of the homoeopath, which is a lengthy and expensive process, or for the process of manufacturing to be exempt from the legislation as outlined in Chapter 6. Most homoeopaths are likely to rely on having exempt status to ensure that their manufacturing processes are legal.

Poisonous substances

It is inherent in the practice of homoeopathy that practitioners will prescribe tinctures of substances that may be poisonous in a more concentrated form. Vigilance is required should they become involved in the production of homoeopathic substances for clients because an error in concentrations could result in poisoning or injury. Adverse events (possibly unrelated to the homoeopathic substances) may occur at the same time a client is undertaking a course of treatment by a homoeopath, so good records of the substances used should be kept. This will aid any investigation of the possible cause of this event in relation to the practitioner.

Adverse reactions

Part of the healing process will often involve a worsening of symptoms before healing occurs. Practitioners should warn of this possibility before beginning treatment.

Goods and Services Tax (GST)

Homoeopathy does not enjoy exempt status under the GST legislation. While this status continues, practitioners registered for this tax will need to recover GST on fees and substances supplied to clients and then remit this amount to the Commissioner for Taxation (refer to page 221).

Acupuncture

Because acupuncture is the only discipline that routinely requires the piercing of a client's skin, some very specific issues arise.

BOX 7.8

Action plan

- Use only non-reusable acupuncture needles.
- Carefully consider the need for consent to treatment.
- Take great care in the use of moxibustion.

Infection control

Refer to pages 84 and 89 for a discussion of required infection-control procedures. A practitioner should use only new single-use acupuncture needles, as any localised infection around a puncture point would raise the issue of whether this infection was caused by an inadequately sterilised needle. Should a client contract hepatitis, HIV or some other infectious illness, a question may arise as to whether this infection was caused by some breach of sterilisation procedures by the acupuncturist. The exclusive use of single-use needles would place the practitioner in a strong position to deal with this issue. The Chinese Medical Board of Australia provides for specific 'Infection prevention and control guidelines for acupuncture practice' which can be found at https://www.chinesemedicineboard.gov.au/Codes-Guidelines/Infection-prevention.aspx (accessed 29 October 2021).

The Board has adopted the National Health and Medical Research Council's (NHMRC) Australian Guidelines for the Prevention and Control of Infection in Healthcare (2019). In addition, the expectation is that all registered acupuncturists must comply with the NHMRC Guidelines, the Chinese Medical Board of Australia Guidelines, and relevant state, territory and local government requirements that apply to their place of business.

Consent to treatment and risks of treatment

Skin piercing

Acupuncture will usually involve the piercing of the skin, and the pain and discomfort associated with that process, so consent to treatment is important. Although complementary medicine will often involve touching or the application of force to a client, the process of piercing the skin may create fears, uncertainties and sensitivity in some clients. Many will understand the basic procedures involved in acupuncture, but this should not be assumed.

To avoid an argument that proper consent was not obtained before treatment, a practitioner should carefully indicate the process involved, such as the necessity to pierce the skin, the time involved, and any pain or discomfort that is likely to ensue. To quell any unnecessary fears, advise clients that single-use needles will be used.

The practice of acupuncture is generally very safe, but any risks of treatment, such as infection at the insertion site or fainting, should be discussed fully or details provided as part of a written document reviewed and signed by a client. Because of the risk of fainting and consequent serious injury, it is important to treat clients on a table rather than standing, and advise them of any risk of fainting on alighting from the table.

Moxibustion

This is a common technique used by practitioners. The process of burning herbs in close proximity to a client's skin has obvious risks. Practitioners should be aware that it would be difficult to resist a claim that negligence had occurred if burning or injury were caused during such a treatment.

Cupping

This technique may cause bruising. A warning about this should be given prior to treatment.

Traditional Chinese medicine

BOX 7.9
___

Action plan

- Avoid using terms that suggest you are a medical doctor.
- Make sure that *Therapeutic Goods Act* requirements are satisfied in relation to pre-scribing herbs.
- Take steps to avoid adverse or unexpected reactions caused by incompatibility of herbs and potions with pharmaceuticals.
- Take steps to secure herbs that are unadulterated.

Therapeutic Goods Act

Practitioners should ensure that their practice incorporates the types of procedures and activities that secure exempt status or satisfy the provisions of the TGA in some other way. Although currently there are limited controls and standards on Chinese herbs, this may change as the legislative regime begins to incorporate further safeguards in relation to the supply of these substances by practitioners (refer to Chapter 6).

Incompatibility with pharmaceuticals

Many Chinese herbs have a very strong impact on the metabolism. For this reason, practitioners need to be aware of the possibility of negative side effects that may result from the herbs, individually and in combination with pharmaceuticals. Some herbs may exaggerate, inhibit or change the effect of pharmaceutical products. A practitioner should ask clients whether they are currently taking any medication.

Practitioners should advise clients of the effect that prescribed herbs and other substances may have on this medication and assess the risks involved. If there is a possibility of an adverse reaction, the client should either be advised of the possible consequences or the substances should not be given without medical advice. In no situation should a practitioner advise a client to stop medication prescribed by a medical doctor. Practitioners should always bear in mind that many clients would not feel free to discuss the treatment they are receiving from the practitioner with their medical doctor.

Quality of herbs and substances

Refer to the discussion in Chapter 6 dealing with the potential liability for the prescribing of adulterated or impure substances as part of clinical practice. It is clearly very important that practitioners source the substances used in their practice from high-quality sources. It is important to ensure that the substance provided to clients:

- is the substance it is represented to be (e.g. it is the specific fresh herb from a particular locality)
- has the represented healing qualities
- is not adulterated in any way by harmful chemicals or substances (e.g. herbs adulterated with aconite), and
- is given with clear instructions as to dosage, preparation or shelf life (if there is ambiguity in these instructions, they may be interpreted against the practitioner).

Scheduling of medicines and poisons

Chinese medicine practitioners may wish to use certain substances that fall within the category of scheduled medicines or poisons. The Chinese Medicine Board of Australia has provided a list of those Chinese herbs and their appropriate use by registered practitioners in the Chinese herbs listed in Standard for the Uniform Scheduling of Medicines and Poisons (June 2021).[27]

Patient records

Chinese medicine practitioners need to consider clause 8.3 of the AHPRA Code of Conduct to understand minimum standards for clinical record-keeping that may be important in proceedings for professional conduct. See https://www.ahpra.gov.au/Publications/Code-of-conduct.aspx.

Advertising for Chinese medicine practitioners[28]

Note the guidelines above at pages 166–167 about general codes and guidelines. Below is some specific information for Chinese medicine:

- Chinese medicine examples of non-compliant advertising: https://www.ahpra.gov.au/Publications/Advertising-hub/Resources-for-advertisers/Chinese-medicine-examples.aspx
- Position statement on Chinese medicine practitioners making therapeutic claims in advertising: https://www.chinesemedicineboard.gov.au/Codes-Guidelines/Position-statements/therapeutic-claims-in-advertising.aspx

Other significant Chinese medicine guidelines

- Professional capabilities for Chinese medicine practitioners
- Guidelines for safe practice of Chinese herbal medicine[29]
- Infection prevention and control guidelines for acupuncture practice

Herbal medicine

Herbalists practise a profession that has had a place in healing throughout history. They prescribe a variety of herbal substances, including traditional Chinese herbs and Australian native herbs, for a wide variety of conditions. This modality may be practised in association with naturopathy or other health modalities.

BOX 7.10

Action plan

- Ensure that *Therapeutic Goods Act* requirements are satisfied in relation to prescribing herbs.
- Take steps to avoid adverse or unexpected reactions to substances such as echinacea or caused by incompatibility of herbs with pharmaceuticals.

Therapeutic Goods Act

The therapeutic effect of many herbal substances may be well known, based on their long use. The TGA provisions should always be borne in mind when administering herbs to clients (refer to Chapter 6).

Adverse reactions

One important consideration for practitioners should be the possibility of adverse reactions to herbal substances. Refer to page 183–184, where the potential liability for susceptible clients is discussed. The possibility of incompatibility with pharmaceutical substances should also be an important consideration.

Yoga

Yoga Australia describes yoga as follows:

> Generally, it is recognised as an ancient system of philosophies, principles and practices derived from the Vedic tradition of India and the Himalayas, more than 2500 years ago. It is a system that recognises the multi-dimensional nature of the human person, and primarily relates to the nature and workings of the mind, based on experiential practice and self-enquiry. Yoga cultivates health and wellbeing (physical, emotional, mental and social) through the regular practice of a range of many different techniques, including postures and movement, breath awareness and breathing exercises, relaxation and concentration, self-inquiry and meditation.[30]

Yoga has many aspects that relate to spiritual and personal growth issues; however, there are some potential legal issues that can arise for yoga practitioners that should be understood beyond the general concepts suggested in this book.

Instructions to clients

Yoga exercises may involve movements with which clients are unfamiliar, especially those new to the practice. Good instruction should be given to clients about how to perform the exercises or movements while under direct instruction, including certain information if it is likely that they may be using these techniques outside the yoga class or instruction. An instructor should carefully consider the capacities of the clients before instruction and counsel care in performing movements beyond their normal range of movement without due preparation. If a client was to perform a movement or exercise and suffer injury, there is a possibility of liability for the yoga instructor if it is considered that the duty of care that would apply to the instructor has been breached and this breach caused the injury and damages have arisen. For this reason, careful instruction, demonstration, supervision and adjustment of practice to deal with potentially dangerous activities and, if possible, written instructions (especially for non-supervised activity) should be provided. It would be good practice to advise a client to stop the practice if pain is felt or the exercise is beyond the physical ability of the client.

Warnings of risks

If a potential risk of yoga includes the possibility of causing pain during or after yoga, then this should be advised. Clients should be asked to consider any injury, disability or sickness that may impact on how they approach their yoga practice. Consideration should be given to discussing potential known risks of yoga.

Holistic counselling

There are many types of counselling involving registered psychologists or unregistered counsellors.

Restricted title

Only registered psychologists are entitled to use the term 'psychologist' under the terms of the National Law. A non-registered counsellor is not entitled to use that title, name, initial, symbol, word or description, sign or device, or another term that, having regard to the circumstances in which it is taken or used, may suggest that the person is a registered psychologist.

Confidentiality and privacy

The discussion about confidentiality on pages 49–52 is very apt for counsellors, as the nature of the practice inevitably involves discussing private personal, financial and health issues with clients and, although this is an issue for all health practitioners, it should be at the front of mind for all counsellors. Any release of confidential information should only occur with the consent of the client or for the other exceptions discussed above at pages 50–51. Associated with confidentiality are the statutory requirements to preserve privacy in relation to health information.

Relationships with clients

Forming a relationship with a client is an issue that arises for psychologists and psychiatrists, and is a common basis for professional misconduct hearings—caused no doubt by the inherent personal connections that may arise from the process of counselling. The violation of boundaries must be avoided, as it has the potential to cause considerable psychological injury to vulnerable clients. Courts and professional tribunals tend to be very severe in those cases involving psychologists, psychiatrists and counsellors for this reason.

Abandonment

The closeness of the counselling process suggests that it is appropriate professional practice to provide proper notice, assistance and information in finding a replacement counsellor if a practitioner is obliged to terminate the counselling relationship or the practitioner is leaving practice through sickness or retirement or is moving or on vacation. Clause B.11 of the Australian Psychological Society (APS) Code of Ethics (adopted by the Psychology Board of Australia) provides some guidance on this issue. Refer to pages 117–118 on the professional and legal issues involved with this issue.

Notes

1 https://www.ahpra.gov.au/Publications/Advertising-hub/Advertising-guidelines-and-other-guidance/Advertising-guidelines.aspx (accessed 28 October 2021).
2 ahpra.gov.au/Publications/Advertising-hub.aspx (accessed 28 October 2021); https://www.ahpra.gov.au/Publications/Advertising-hub/Resources-for-advertisers.aspx (accessed 19 February 2022).
3 https://www.ahpra.gov.au/Publications/Code-of-conduct.aspx (accessed 19 February 2022).
4 https://www.ahpra.gov.au/Publications/Social-media-guidance.aspx (accessed 28 October 2021).
5 https://www.ahpra.gov.au/Notifications/mandatorynotifications/Mandatory-notifications.aspx (accessed 28 October 2021).
6 *Rosenberg v Cahill* 492 A.2d 371 (NJ 1985).
7 J.D. Harrison, *Chiropractic Practice Liability: A Practical Guide to Successful Risk Management*, International Chiropractors Association, Arlington, VA, 1990, Chapter 19.
8 A. Terrett, 'Misuse of the Literature by Medical Authors in Discussing Spinal Manipulative Therapy' (1995) 18 *Journal of Manipulative and Physiological Therapeutics* 4 at 203; *Forder v Hutchinson* [2005] VSCA 281 (osteopath).
9 A.M. Kleynhans, 'Complications of and Contraindications to Spinal Manipulative Therapy', in Scott Haldeman (ed.), *Principles and Practice of Chiropractic*, McGraw-Hill, New York, 2005, Chapter 16; A.G.J. Terrett & A.M. Kleynhans, 'Cerebrovascular Complications of Manipulations', in Haldeman, *Principles and Practice of Chiropractic*, pp. 579–98; Maurizio Paciaroni & Julien Bogousslavsky, 'Cerebrovascular Complications of Neck Manipulation' (2009) 61 *European Neurology* 112–118.
10 Kleynhans, 'Complications of and Contraindications to Spinal Manipulative Therapy', p. 377.
11 Terrett & Kleynhans, 'Cerebrovascular Complications of Manipulations', p. 580.
12 Kleynhans, 'Complications of and Contraindications to Spinal Manipulative Therapy', pp. 378–9.
13 Chiropractic Board of Australia, 'Code of Conduct for Chiropractors', cl. 3.6. https://www.chiropracticboard.gov.au/Codes-guidelines/Code-of-conduct.aspx (accessed 28 October 2021).

14 https://www.ahpra.gov.au/Publications/Code-of-conduct.aspx.
15 Chiropractic Board of Australia, Position statement, March 2019, Interim policy on spinal manipulation for infants and young children, 2.
16 https://www.chiropracticboard.gov.au/Codes-guidelines/Position-statements/Interim-policy-on-spinal-manipulation.aspx (accessed 17 December 2021).
17 https://www.ahpra.gov.au/Publications/Advertising-hub/Resources-for-advertisers/Chiropractic-examples.aspx (accessed 17 December 2021).
18 *Chiropractic Board of Australia v Shanahan* [2017] SAHPT 9 [53].
19 www.chiropracticboard.gov.au/News/2018-08-28-Chiropractor-reprimanded.aspx (accessed 28 October 2021).
20 https://www.ahpra.gov.au/News/2018-02-06-ahpra-successfully-prosecutes-fake-qld-chir.aspx (accessed 28 October 2021).
21 [2004] SADC 190 (22 December 2004).
22 Paul Finch, 'The Motivation of Massage Therapy Students to Enter Professional Education', 26 *Medical Teacher* 8, 729–731.
23 Sarah Oerton, 'Bodywork Boundaries: Power, Politics and Professionalism in Therapeutic Massage' (2004) 11 *Gender Work and Organization*, 543–565.
24 Ibid, 550.
25 http://www.atms.com.au/visageimages/Policies%20%26%20Conduct/ATMS-OFFICIAL-POLICIES-Information_July2015.pdf (accessed 29 October 2021).
26 https://www.massagemyotherapy.com.au/Consumers/Code-of-Conduct-and-Complaints/During-Treatment-What-to-expect-and-Appropriate-Draping (accessed 29 October 2021); http://www.amt.org.au/downloads/practice-resources/AMT-code-of-practice-final.pdf (accessed 29 October 2021).
27 https://www.chinesemedicineboard.gov.au/Codes-Guidelines/Guidelines-for-safe-practice.aspx (accessed 29 October 2021).
28 https://www.chinesemedicineboard.gov.au/Codes-Guidelines/Advertising-a-regulated-health-service.aspx (accessed 29 October 2021).
29 https://www.chinesemedicineboard.gov.au/Codes-Guidelines/Guidelines-for-safe-practice.aspx (accessed 29 October 2021).
30 www.yogaaustralia.org.au/what-is-yoga (accessed 17 December 2021).

8 Setting up a practice

Most practitioners will choose to enter private practice. You need to think about the appropriate legal structure for your practice and the legal issues that confront a practitioner as a small business proprietor. If you are thinking of a small part-time practice at home, you may need only to register a business name and operate as a sole trader. A more sophisticated practice might require you to team up with another person or persons in a partnership. If you expect to be earning substantial fees, perhaps the use of a company and/or trust structure might be advisable. Some people are prepared to build up their practice from scratch, while many will choose to buy into a partnership or purchase an existing business.

Whichever type of practice is contemplated, it is important to understand the available options for trading structures so as to maximise flexibility, lessen the incidence of taxation and, if possible, protect against legal liability. Commercial reality suggests the need to carefully consider the practice's legal and financial structure, the issues involved in buying a practice and those related to undertaking a commercial lease or running a practice from home. This chapter will deal with many significant issues, but individual professional advice should always be sought from an accountant and/or lawyer where appropriate.

BOX 8.1

Action plan

Business plan

An important first step for a practitioner contemplating setting up a practice is to prepare a business plan. The business plan is to satisfy yourself that your proposal is viable, to focus your efforts and, if necessary, to convince financiers that your business is worth supporting financially. A business plan requires some time and thought and may be improved by input from an accountant or other professional. When preparing a business plan, think about:

- Strategic plan. Where are you now and where do you hope to be in the short, medium and long term?
- Marketing. How will your clients know about you and what you do?
- Clientele profile. What types of people will use your services?
- Market research. What is the market you are targeting? Can you supply their needs? Are you siting the business in the correct geographical location?

DOI: 10.4324/9781003195931-8

- Appointment of a lawyer and accountant. Who is the appropriate legal and accounting person who will have the necessary expertise to provide appropriate input into your practice?
- Business name and intellectual property (e.g. trademarks and designs).
- Leasing of premises. What type, where, how big? Are the premises legally compliant for the intended practice?
- Human capital. The need for technical, administrative and professional staff.
- Finance needs, accounting systems, computer equipment, cash flow projections.
- Strengths and weaknesses of your business and competitors.
- Competitive advantage.
- Expected economic and market conditions.

BOX 8.2

Professional requirements

- Do you have or need appropriate formal education and/or training for the intended practice?
- Seek membership of the appropriate professional body or bodies.
- Obtain professional registration (if required under the National Law).
- Read and understand the relevant code of ethics or statutory provisions.
- Maintain an appropriate level of professional indemnity insurance.
- Obtain a provider number for health fund refunds (if applicable).

BOX 8.3

Trading

- Obtain registration or listing of goods used in the practice under the *Therapeutic Goods Act* and/or ensure exemption applicable to your practice.
- Obtain a Yellow Pages entry and other advertising sources, and establish a website, making sure that advertising is not misleading or in breach of applicable statutes.
- Arrange signage in accordance with local authority and professional requirements.
- Negotiate appropriate financing arrangements.
- Implement accounting procedures, including GST requirements (if necessary).

Business names

All businesses, unless exempt, must register a business name through the Australian Securities and Investments Commission (ASIC).[1] Very useful information about how to approach creating a business name is provided by this Commonwealth government link: https://asic.gov.au/for-business/registering-a-business-name.

Business name registration is not required in New Zealand but a business can apply for a New Zealand Business Number (NZBN).

Purpose of legislation

The policy behind the Australian business name legislation is intended to[2]:

- 'ensure that business names that are undesirable (for example, because they are offensive) are not registered'
- 'identify the entity and how the entity may be contacted'; and
- avoid confusion among the public in relation to identical or similar names.

Names requiring registration

Any business name must be registered except in the case of:

- a person trading only under their own names (e.g. 'Philip John Wade')
- a family name with the initials for the given name or names (e.g. 'P.J. Wade')
- a family name with a combination of given names and initials (e.g. 'Philip J. Wade')

Thus a practitioner trading as a sole trader under the business name John Smith Naturopath or Jane Brown Chiropractor would need to register the business name as the business name includes a description of the modality. The same would apply to the use of J. Smith Naturopath or J. Brown Chiropractor.

If you trade as a partnership or in association, business name registration is needed unless the business name reflects only the full names or family names and initials of all persons trading under that business name. For example, a two-person firm that was trading as J. Jones and M. Brown Naturopaths would require registration. If the name used does not relate to the names of the persons carrying on business (e.g. Positive Health Natural Therapies Clinic), or if the name used is not the full name or surname and initials of the practitioners (e.g. Jones and Brown Naturopaths), then registration will be necessary.

Registration requires lodgement of a registration form and fee, and annual renewal. Registration will occur only after ASIC has established that the business name is not identical or so similar to another registered business name or company name as to cause confusion. An application for a business name requires the applicant to provide an Australian Business Number (ABN). When registration of the business name has occurred, the business name must be displayed prominently at the premises where the business is carried on. Business name registration is not required where the entity is a corporation and the name is incorporated in the corporate name.

Legal status

A business name can be protected by legal action but it does not create a separate legal entity that can sue or be sued. Any liability for debts or other obligations accrues to the person or entity trading under that business name.

Passing off

The reputation of a business can be protected under the common law tort of 'passing off'. This remedy applies if a business is representing itself to be another business and this causes damage. Passing off could occur if, for example, an established business trades as Natural Health Therapies Clinic and another business called Natural Health Therapies Centre begins trading in the vicinity. This might be considered passing off, especially if the business uses similar signage and advertising to attract the clientele of the other trader, and causes damage to the original business. This may also be an offence under the relevant *Business Names Register Act* if the second trader does not have a registered business name.

Trademarks

A registered business name is not the same as having a trademark. If you want to protect a logo, distinctive name, brand or device against its use by someone else, you should consider registering a trademark, as this would permit you to obtain a monopoly on its use. The process of registering a trademark is more complex and more expensive than that of registering a business name. You could ask a patent attorney to attend to that task on your own behalf. IP Australia provides the requirements (https://www.ipaustralia.gov.au/trade-marks).

Medicare and health insurance

Medicare, the national government health system, makes limited provision for a chiropractor or osteopath to provide Medicare-funded health services through a referral by a general practitioner under a GP Management Plan and Team Care Arrangement or, in the case of a person resident in an aged care facility, as part of a multidisciplinary care plan. These arrangements entitle the chiropractor or osteopath to a Medicare benefit for a maximum of five services per patient each calendar year based upon services directly related to a patient's chronic medical condition and identified in their care plan. A general practitioner determines whether the patient's chronic medical condition would benefit from these health services. If the chiropractor or osteopath accepts the Medicare benefit as full payment for the service, there is no other payment; otherwise the patient pays the difference between the fee charged and the Medicare rebate. There is an obligation for the chiropractor or osteopath to report back to the referring GP.[3]

From 1 April 2019 the Federal government excluded from private health insurance sixteen modalities: Alexander technique, aromatherapy, Bowen therapy, buteyko, feldenkrais, western herbalism, homeopathy, iridology, kinesiology, naturopathy, pilates, reflexology, rolfing, shiatsu, tai chi and yoga. Remedial massage/myotherapy, exercise physiology, Chinese medicine, and acupuncture were not impacted by this change. The Natural Therapies Review 2019–20 under the Natural Therapies Review Expert Advisory Panel is currently reviewing that decision to determine if this change should be repealed.

Treatment provided by a complementary medicine practitioner is eligible for coverage by private health insurance if the practitioner is duly registered, such as applies to chiropractic, osteopathy and Chinese medicine for the treatment contemplated by that registration or remedial massage/myotherapy and exercise physiology.

Trading structures

Choosing a suitable structure

The most appropriate trading structure will depend on the intentions of the person or persons involved in the enterprise and the nature of the practice. This chapter will describe four options: sole trader, partnership, company and trust.

BOX 8.4

Action plan

Trading structure

- Obtain advice from a lawyer and/or accountant as to an appropriate trading structure, including relevant documentation.
- Choose an appropriate trading structure and ensure that proper documentation is completed.
- Register a business name if required.

BOX 8.5

Practice tip: Criteria for choice of structure

The answers to these questions will impact upon which trading structure should be preferred:

- Will the practice be for one or a number of modalities? Will it involve non-professional activities such as a bookshop or health-food store attached to a naturopathy clinic?
- Is the practice intended to be full time or part time?
- Will others, such as a spouse, children or other practitioners, be involved in the practice?
- What financing arrangements are necessary?
- What is the intended duration of the practice?
- What level of income is expected from the practice?
- Do you expect the practice to make a loss in the first year (or longer)?
- Do you think you will need to introduce new participants?
- Do professional requirements allow you to incorporate?

Assessment criteria

The four options will be assessed generally on the basis of the following criteria: nature of structure, cost to set up and maintain, tax liability, simplicity, legal liability, ability to sell the entire business, ability to admit new participants and control.

Sole trader

This structure is appropriate for many practitioners because of its low set-up and maintenance costs. The small scale of many practices means that the tax disadvantages initially may not be of great importance. If a full-time and sophisticated practice is contemplated, other structures may provide substantial advantages over sole trading.

Nature of structure

A sole trader is a person who trades as himself/herself without partners, shareholders or directors.

Simplicity

A sole trader is the simplest business structure. It involves the least administrative burden and legal regulation, and there is little continuing administration attached to the structure itself. The normal administrative and legal requirements include:

- maintaining an Australian Business Number (ABN) and considering whether to register for the Goods and Services Tax (GST)
- maintaining a basic set of accounts and records
- pay-as-you-go (PAYG) tax in instalments for yourself and any employees
- tax returns
- licences from state or local government. Australian Business Licence and Information Service (ABLIS)[4] provides access to the licences, regulations and approvals that may arise for your business.
- insurance for premises and professional indemnity
- finance arrangements (e.g. bank loan)
- lease payments for premises or equipment
- employee superannuation and workers' compensation (if any), and
- business name registration (if required).

Costs of set-up and maintenance

The costs involved in set-up are limited. A sole trader can simply start practice with little formal documentation or structure. Registering for an ABN and the GST is dealt with below. If the sole trader has employees, there are some formalities. Employers must register with the Australian Taxation Office (ATO), and are required to withhold tax from salary or wages paid to employees and contribute superannuation payments and workers' compensation payments, and keep proper records.

Tax liability

ADVANTAGES

There are several tax advantages of being a sole trader:

- Losses can be offset against income from other sources to reduce tax liability.
- On commencement of trading, the initial payment of tax can be delayed for a period after taxable income is earned, because pay as you go (PAYG) tax is not payable until then.
- Capital gains tax discounting of 50 per cent may be available.

DISADVANTAGES

Tax liability may not be an important issue where the practice does not derive sufficient income to pay a significant amount of income tax. The tax disadvantages are that PAYG instalments will be payable on net income. Although PAYG income tax may not be paid during the first year of trading, on lodgement of the first tax return, the ATO will advise the sole trader of an instalment rate. This is then applied to the trader's quarterly income or, when the tax payable is less than the specified threshold

$8,000, to the annual income. In practice, this will mean paying, at about the same time, tax on the first year's trading plus a quarterly or yearly instalment of tax for the following year. This can have a negative effect on the cash flow in the second year unless proper provision is made for such payment.

A sole trader cannot take advantage of an income-splitting strategy to use the tax-free threshold and lower rates on tax that is available in other structures, unless family members are employed in the business. Where family members are employees, they must be paid a reasonable wage for work performed and not an inflated amount.

In some cases a person may not be obliged to reveal profits made from an activity that is not a business but might be considered a hobby. This will not be applicable to most complementary medicine practices but it may arise in the case of a limited part-time practice. There are no fixed rules that apply, but this might arise where the revenue from the business is not substantial. The factors that suggest your practice is not a hobby are:

- You have decided to commence a business and have registered a business name or obtained an Australian Business Name.
- You are seeking to make a profit from the activity.
- Your activity involves repeating similar types of activities such as the regular provision of massage therapy treatments.
- The size of the activity is consistent with other businesses in the industry.
- If the activity is based on planning, it involves organisation and is characterised by normal business-like features such as keeping business records and books; holding a separate business bank account; operating from business premises; having a licence for the premises; or having qualifications relevant to the activity.[5]

Legal liability

A sole trader's legal liability is unlimited. Any debts of the business are those of the sole trader personally, and creditors have recourse to the assets of the sole trader. For this reason, public liability and professional indemnity insurance should be maintained.

Ability to sell

A sole trader is not limited in the sale of the practice. The sale will require legal documentation that is best dealt with by a lawyer and may involve the input of an accountant. An important aspect of the value of the practice will be the goodwill component, which is calculated based on the reputation created by the practitioner and reflected in the income generated by the business.

Ability to admit a new participant

If it is intended to share profits with another practitioner, a formal partnership structure may be advisable. If one or more practitioners intend to trade as sole traders from the same premises, a partnership may be created if it involves a joint enterprise with the view to profit, even if the parties do not actually intend to create a partnership.

Control

The sole trader has the sole responsibility to determine the future direction of the business. Sole traders don't have the advantage of assistance and advice from partners or directors, so they should seek advice from accountants and lawyers on important decisions to ensure that all legal requirements are satisfied and business implications are understood.

Partnerships

A partnership allows the pooling of resources and skills, and is comparatively simple to administer. The major disadvantages of this structure are the ability to successfully withdraw from the structure and the potential liability for the acts of partners.

Nature of structure

A partnership or firm is a business organisation of at least two persons who, in common, are carrying on business with a view to profit. The advantage of a partnership is that it pools the collective assets, skill, knowledge and knowhow of the partners for mutual benefit.

Simplicity

A partnership can be created with a minimum of complex documentation. There is no need for any specific formalities to create a partnership, as this may be implied by carrying on business in common with a view to profit. This may create a partnership even when the parties did not intend that this would occur.

Practitioners contemplating a partnership are better protected by entry into a written partnership agreement that carefully expresses the mutual obligations and entitlements of the partners. Without a partnership agreement, the common law and the relevant *Partnership Act* for that jurisdiction in Australia or New Zealand will govern the relationship between the parties. This may provide results the partners did not intend.

By agreeing on issues such as profit-sharing, retirement, dissolution, provision for drawings, salaries and dispute resolution, any conflict may be averted or controlled. The types of matter that should be dealt with in a partnership agreement are:

* the names of the partners and the business name
* the nature of the business (e.g. will it involve chiropractic, naturopathy or massage therapy?)
* the duration of the partnership (e.g. will it be for three or five years or unlimited?)
* the capital being introduced by each partner
* accounting details
* the authority of partners to bind the others
* how profits are to be distributed (i.e. is it equal or unequal?)
* provisions for drawings from profit by partners
* provision for salaries
* interest on capital

- provision should a partner die or enter bankruptcy
- retirement of partners, and
- valuation of partnership business on death, retirement or dissolution.

Costs of set-up and maintenance

A partnership agreement should be drafted by a lawyer. Although the set-up cost of a partnership is higher than that of a sole trader, this cost is not prohibitive and reflects the need to clearly spell out the mutual obligations of partners. A partnership will likely need to register and maintain a business name, set up a partnership bank account, print stationery in the partnership name, register for an ABN and GST (if the turnover is $75,000 or above), register as an employer with the ATO if employees are involved, obtain a tax file number for the partnership, and set up superannuation arrangements and workers' compensation for any employees.

Tax liability

The tax liability of partnerships is similar to that of sole traders, with the advantage that partnerships, especially between family members, allow income-splitting to occur. A member of the family who is a partner can be paid a reasonable salary or percentage of the profit to lower the total income of each partner. This allows each family member, as a partner, to be subject to lower tax rates and take advantage of any tax-free threshold.

A partnership lodges a separate tax return, though partners pay income tax separately. Because partners are taxed as individuals, they may also be able to claim a 50 per cent discount on capital gains tax. The same PAYG rules apply as for sole traders. The nature of partnership taxation makes it better for assets to be owned by the individual partners and not in the partnership. Assets can be leased to the partnership.

Legal liability and control

One major risk of partnerships (discussed in more detail below) is the potential liability for any negligent acts and debts created in the name of the partnership, including debts incurred by a partner acting outside the express authority of the partnership. Unless otherwise provided for in the partnership deed, ordinary decisions of the partnership are by majority. A change to the nature of the business or the introduction of new partners requires the agreement of all partners.

Ability to sell and to admit new participants

A partner can sell his or her interest in the partnership to a third party. Normally, this would require the consent of the other partners. Partnership deeds often require a retiring partner to first offer their share to the continuing partners.

The value of the retiring partner's share of the partnership business is a common source of dispute between partners. The difficulty of withdrawing from a partnership without dispute confirms the importance of choosing compatible partners and specifying clear and workable arrangements in the partnership agreement with regard to retirement, dealing with how the value of the retiring partner's interest should be calculated.

Relations of partners to outsiders

The *Partnership Act* confirms that a partner will bind the other partners when acting in the business of the partnership. This authority may be limited by the partnership agreement, thereby limiting the liability of partners where the person with whom he or she deals is aware of that limitation.

More significantly, if a partner has no authority to enter into a transaction, an act carried on in the usual way of the business of the firm is binding on the other partners unless the person with whom he or she contracted knew that the partner had no authority or did not know they were a partner. In this way, liability can arise for partners where another partner acts without authority. This means that a partner may bind the other partners—for example, in the purchase of commercial premises for the practice—even if he or she has no such authority. Partners are also bound by the torts such as negligence of partners committed in the course of the firm's business or with their authority. As a result, if a partner is negligent in their practice, this liability would usually attach to all the partners. Ideally, any liability will be covered by professional indemnity insurance, discussed on pages 225–230.

Incorporated companies

The use of an incorporated company is worthwhile when a full-time practice is contemplated and it is likely that substantial fees will be generated. This structure provides advantages for taxation and superannuation. Unless the expected income is sufficient to obtain these benefits, the costs of set-up and administration may not be justified. There are complicated ATO provisions in relation to taxation of incorporated practices which require advice from an accountant or lawyer.

Nature of structure

TYPES OF COMPANY

Among the various types of corporate structures available, most professionals will choose a small proprietary company limited by shares. A company is created in Australia by incorporation under the *Corporations Act 2001* and in New Zealand under the *Companies Act 1993*. On incorporation, the company becomes a separate legal entity and can enter into contracts, and sue and be sued.

FEATURES OF A COMPANY

The primary features of a company are:

* shareholders (there must be at least one)
* directors (the persons who are obliged to make decisions for the company in its best interests), and
* constitution (the document that sets out the objects and aims of the company).

Simplicity

Companies have a greater level of complexity than the sole trader and partnership structures because of the complex interplay between shareholders and directors, and the requirements of the *Corporations Act 2001* in Australia and the *Companies Act 1993* in New Zealand. This suggests the need for advice from lawyers and/or accountants.

Costs of set-up and maintenance

The administrative tasks attached to a corporate structure include:

- maintaining a registered office (this will often be a lawyer's or accountant's office)
- keeping detailed accounts to explain transactions and the financial position of the company
- maintaining a register of members and debenture holders
- auditing accounts and financial statements
- formalities in passing resolutions and meetings
- registering for an ABN and GST
- registering as an employer with the ATO
- obtaining a tax file number
- setting up superannuation and workers' compensation arrangements for any employee
- registering a business name (if required), and
- lodgement of annual returns and other documents.

Normally, the services of an accountant and/or lawyer will be required to incorporate a company or for the purchase of an already-incorporated company (shelf company).

Tax liability

There are substantial tax advantages and some disadvantages in using a corporate structure:

ADVANTAGES

- If a company structure is used, a practitioner can be paid a salary and pay tax on a PAYG basis, thereby avoiding the necessity to deal with the requirements of quarterly PAYG instalments.
- Dividend income can be split between family members who are shareholders.
- The use of a superannuation fund to benefit employees can reduce the incidence of taxation.
- For most companies income is taxed at a flat company rate of 25 per cent (in Australia); this may be lower than the normal tax rate under personal income tax rates.
- The company can provide tax-free or low-tax income to shareholders by the use of franked dividends, where the company pre-pays income tax and the shareholder can use these dividends as imputation credits against other income.
- Corporate structure may limit liability.

DISADVANTAGES

- Losses in the company are quarantined. They cannot be offset against other personal income. If you have income from sources outside the company, you are not able to offset company losses against the income received on that separate income.

- There is no tax-free threshold. Income tax is normally levied from the first dollar at a rate of 25 per cent for companies under $50 million in turnover. Accordingly, if the intention is to earn small amounts, there would be little advantage in using this structure as you would not have the advantage of the tax-free threshold available to other taxpayers.
- Dividends must be paid in proportion to shares held. This may not suit the interests of some family members with high incomes.
- The personal discount for capital gains tax does not apply to companies.

Legal liability

In a proprietary limited (Pty Ltd) company, the shareholders are limited in their personal liability to any unpaid amounts on their shares. If a company becomes liable to a debt, a fully paid shareholder has no personal liability for that debt. Limited liability is one major advantage of company structures over partnerships of natural persons, because partners are normally personally liable for all the debts of the business. However, a director of a company may be personally liable for the debts of the company incurred when trading while insolvent or under a personal guarantee given by that director for obligations of the company. This might occur where a company enters a commercial lease and the landlord requires a personal guarantee to enter into this obligation.

Ability to sell

The sale of the practice owned by a company can be achieved by selling all the shares in the company that owns the practice, or by selling on the business owned by the company.

Introduction of new participants

A new participant can be introduced by issuing new shares (subject to the terms of the constitution) or the sale of existing shares in the company. It is possible to enter into a shareholders' agreement that specifies how a retiring or deceased shareholder's interest in the company should be dealt with and valued.

Provision is usually made for shares to be offered first to continuing shareholders. As with partnerships, without prior agreement on the valuation process there is potential for disagreement as to the valuation of the business of the company and/or the shares in the company.

Control

The control and management of the company are in the hands of the directors. In most small, professional corporate structures, the directors will be the shareholders. The shareholders cannot require the directors to take any particular steps, though the members, if unhappy, can vote to remove a director.

Although the directors are not subject to direction by the shareholders, in a general meeting the shareholders have considerable power in some circumstances.

Shareholders can bring an action to stop an act that is grossly unfair to a section of the shareholders (called 'a fraud on the minority') or, where there is oppression or injustice, to wind up the company.

Directors have duties to:

- act bona fide in the interests of the company
- exercise powers for the purpose for which they are conferred
- not to fetter future exercise of their powers
- avoid actual and potential conflicts of interest and duty, and
- act honestly.

Registration for registered health practitioners using a company structure

Registered health practitioners such as chiropractors, osteopaths and Chinese medicine practitioners are not entitled to obtain registration under the name of a company under the National Law, as registration is only possible for an individual. Legal and accounting advice is advisable in relation to income taxation when using a professional service company, as this may be seen to unreasonably lower income tax where predominant income comes from personal services through the personal efforts or skills of the individual professional practitioner.

Trusts

A trading trust may be set up when substantial income is expected from the practice. Distributing income to family members could mean tax savings. A unit trust can also be a practical structure when a practice owned by the trust is distributed among a number of practitioners as unit holders.

Nature of structure

Trusts are devices primarily for the purposes of reducing liability for income tax and asset protection. The trust is usually created by a written trust deed in which a settlor vests a nominal amount on a trustee on trust for beneficiaries. After the establishment of the trust, further assets are vested in the trust either by the trustee starting to trade or by a transfer of business to the trustee. This structure is called a trading trust. A trust is not a separate legal entity. The trustee can be a natural person but is more commonly a proprietary limited liability company.

DISCRETIONARY TRUST

The most common form of trust is a discretionary trust, which caters for estate planning within a family grouping. The trustee distributes income that is derived by the trust to the beneficiaries, as the trustee in its discretion deems appropriate. In a discretionary trust, the beneficiaries will normally be widely defined to include spouses, children and grandchildren of the settlor or of the family involved in the trust. This structure allows maximum flexibility for the income-splitting that is the primary reason for using this structure.

FIXED TRUST

Here, the income of the trust is distributed to named beneficiaries in fixed proportions. This structure does not allow the same flexibility in taxation planning. A common type of fixed trust is a unit trust.

A unit trust is usually used where a number of people wish to pool resources based on a proportion of the total number of units in the unit trust. The unit trust has a settlor and trustee (normally a corporate trustee controlled by the unit holders) and a specified number of units in the trust. It might have four units distributed to four different stated beneficiaries, or any other appropriate variation. The beneficiaries may be individuals, companies or other unit trusts or discretionary trusts.

Simplicity

The fixed trust is the most complex of the structures discussed as it involves a trust, trustee (usually corporate), beneficiaries and attendant complexities in taxation and administration.

Ability to sell and to introduce new members

If the unit trust deed permits, units can be transferred to new unit holders or new units can be issued. Extra beneficiaries can be introduced into a discretionary trust, though this may have significant stamp duty consequences.

Costs of set-up and maintenance

This type of structure will involve the set-up and maintenance of a corporate trustee, a trust and a register of beneficiaries, all of which have somewhat complex taxation, legal and accounting requirements. Accordingly, this structure will be more expensive in terms of set-up and maintenance than the other structures discussed here, as more legal and accounting advice will be required on commencement and on a continuing basis.

Tax liability

A trust structure will normally maximise tax advantages but will add some complexity to tax arrangements. Trusts have the advantages available to companies and are taxed as companies. Imputation credits are available for trust dividends.

The primary purpose of the use of trusts is the ability to split income among family members, including children. It provides a great deal of flexibility in the way that the share of income is varied in each tax year. The tax law governing trusts is extremely complex and it is vital that you consult a tax adviser before setting up this structure.

Legal liability

The law in relation to both the legal liability of trustees and beneficiaries, and the entitlements of creditors is complex. Normally, a trustee can recover from trust assets any liability undertaken within the terms of the trust. A well-drafted trust deed will limit the liability of beneficiaries for the debts of the trust.

Ability to deal with interest

The corporate trustee may be one of a number of shareholders of a company that owns the practice. A transfer of the share owned by the trustee in the company owning the practice could complete a transfer of a share of the practice.

If a discretionary trust is the sole owner of the shares in the company owning the practice, or if the discretionary trust owns the practice directly, a transfer of the business would only be practical by a transfer of the business itself.

Control

The trustee, who is obliged to act in accordance with the trust for the benefit of the beneficiaries, controls the trust. If the trustee acts improperly, they may be subject to an action by the beneficiaries to recover monies, or a court order that the trustee act according to the trust.

Leasing premises

Many practitioners will choose to lease or sub-lease premises. A commercial lease is a legal obligation requiring careful thought and negotiation. This section will discuss a number of important matters to consider before entering a lease. Also discussed are particular requirements for specific modalities, such as massage and acupuncture, and the question of occupier's liability.

BOX 8.6

Action plan

Premises and equipment

- Obtain local authority approval, if this is required for the proposed use.
- Ensure conformity with state government, local authority, health, and workplace health and safety requirements. The Australian Business Licence and Information Service (ABLIS) provides access to the licences, regulations and approvals that may arise for your business.
- Negotiate purchase, sub-lease or lease of premises suitable for the intended use.
- Ensure compliance with relevant skin-penetration regulation requirements (if applicable).
- Secure appropriate premises and building, as well as personal, property and public liability insurance policies.
- Make required provision for security and client privacy.
- Purchase equipment, fixtures and fittings that are safe, and obtain proper training in their use.
- Make alterations to leased premises or residence to meet practice requirements.
- Obtain the Australian Performing Right Association Ltd (APRA) licence if you intend to provide music, live performances, videos and so on for your clients.

Lease issues

Consider the following when contemplating a commercial lease.

Term

What is the term of the lease? Six months? One, two, three or five years? Is that term too short or too long? If a practitioner enters a fixed-term lease and later decides to sell, move or cease trading, the tenant must continue paying rent for the balance of the fixed term. A tenant could seek a surrender of the lease (which is unlikely without substantial payment to the landlord) or, with the landlord's consent, assign to a new tenant (an assignee) or sub-lease to a sub-tenant. Many leases may need to be registered with the relevant Land Titles Office to protect the enforceability of the lease against subsequent owners. Your lawyer should provide advice on this matter.

If a lease is assigned, unless the landlord releases the original tenant, the original tenant will often remain contractually bound to the landlord during the remainder of the lease. If the assignee defaults under the lease, the landlord may seek recovery from the original tenant. The original tenant could seek to recover this liability from the assignee.

A sub-lease creates a new landlord–tenant relationship between the tenant and the sub-tenant. The original lease relationship, called 'the head lease', remains. A sub-tenant paying rent to the tenant can contribute all or part of the rent payable under the head lease.

Rent and other payments

OVERALL COST

Check carefully the total payments under the lease. Unlike normal residential leases most commercial leases will expect the tenant to cover outgoings. Outgoings may include:

- rent (some leases include turnover rent, which is based on a percentage of the turnover of the practice), and
- costs of cleaning, rates, land tax and advertising fees.

RENT REVIEWS

There will probably be reviews of rent on the basis of:

- movements in the consumer price index, and
- movements in market rent value.

Some leases state that in no circumstance will rent be lower after a rent review. Even if the market rent declines, the rent payable will not decrease.

Permitted use

The lease will normally specify the permitted use for the premises. Ensure that the intended use:

- is covered by the permitted use clause, as the landlord may be entitled to limit the use to the activities specified, and
- complies with local authority planning provisions.

BOX 8.7

Practice tip: Agreements to lease

The landlord or his or her real estate agent may ask a practitioner to sign a document called an 'agreement to lease' or 'intention to lease'. In some circumstances, this might bind a tenant to a lease before final documentation is finalised. Seek advice from a lawyer before signing this type of document.

A lease that specifies a use that is illegal under local planning provisions may be unenforceable by the landlord and tenant. The permitted use clause should be wide enough to allow some variation in a practice over time. For example, if the usage clause allows only an acupuncture clinic, then any other type of practice would require a variation of this clause to avoid a breach of the lease. This will also limit the permitted practice for any new owner of the business if the lease is assigned or sub-leased unless a broader permitted use clause can be negotiated. It may be preferable to denote the usage clause in general terms, such as 'health services clinic', or even more broadly.

Retail shop leases legislation

Legislation relating to retail shop leases in most states in Australia deals particularly with leases of premises in retail shopping centres and other commercial premises. The legislation may require minimum standards of disclosure and compulsory provisions, as well as providing remedies to tenants. A tenant should seek legal advice regarding how these provisions might affect the lease documentation.

Searches

A lawyer should be employed to complete conveyancing searches to ensure that there are no outstanding notices or requisitions that might hinder the practice.

Default

Provision will be made in the lease for termination on default of the tenant. Default may be non-payment of rent or non-observance of a covenant such as a covenant to repair. The tenant must be given notice before a landlord can terminate a tenancy. These notice provisions normally cannot be excluded.

BOX 8.8

Practice tip

If a tenant is temporarily financially embarrassed and unable to pay rent on time, or there is some misunderstanding about a covenant in a lease, it is usually best to tell the landlord and to negotiate a solution if possible. A lack of information may lead the landlord to assume the worst and to take more drastic steps in relation to the lease.

General issues

- Do the premises comply with health and occupational workplace legislation?
- Do the premises have access to toilets and safe stairways?
- Do the premises have adequate room for treatment and reception of clients?
- Is there adequate parking for clients?
- Are the premises situated where your clients live? Are the premises located in a place where there is undue competition (some localities may be over- or under-serviced)?
- Will the other businesses complement your business? For example, a chiropractic practice may generate business for a massage therapist and vice versa.
- Do the premises provide privacy for clients?

Sub-leasing

Practitioners may choose to sub-lease premises from another practitioner who has a lease from the landlord. The parties to a sub-lease are a landlord/head lessor who grants a head lease to a tenant/lessee. The tenant/lessee then grants a sub-lease to a sub-tenant/sub-lessee.

Sub-leasing may reduce the costs of setting up practice while allowing the practitioner to enjoy some of the advantages of being part of larger premises. The sub-lease may be of the entire premises for the balance of the term of the tenant or may be for part of the leased area.

The landlord has a direct legal relationship with the tenant under the head lease. The landlord has no direct relationship with the sub-tenant unless the head lessor and the sub-tenant enter a contractual arrangement. Rental under the sub-lease will normally be paid to the tenant, who is acting as landlord to the sub-tenant.

The creation of the sub-lease will normally require the consent of the head lessor, otherwise the tenant may be in breach of the terms of the head lease and may be liable in an action for termination of the tenancy. Ensure that the head lease permits sub-leasing and that the landlord consents to the sub-lease.

The landlord may require a formal Consent to Sub-lease document to be prepared, which will establish a direct contractual relationship between the landlord and sub-tenant, which can be enforced in the case of a breach of the lease by the sub-tenant. The head lessor may also require details of the financial viability and experience of the sub-tenant before giving consent if the lease so provides.

Disadvantages of sub-leasing

Some disadvantages of sub-leasing should also be considered.

- *Lack of control.* Subject to the agreement entered into between the tenant and sub-tenant, there may be a lack of control over the leased area because the tenant as the primary user may be more influential with the landlord and with other parties. This may impact upon the sub-tenant's ability to have the premises compliant with legal and/or professional requirements.
- *Subject to head lease.* Although in some states sub-tenants may be protected where the head lease is terminated, the security of tenure is subject to the viability of the

head lease. If the head lease is terminated because of the default of the tenant, this may mean the loss of the sub-lease.

- *Incompatibility.* Consider the compatibility of the tenant and sub-tenant, both in personality and practice modality. The level of noise, smell, or number or type of clients may cause friction that will need to be dealt with by the tenant and sub-tenant.

Any sub-lease arrangement should be documented by a lawyer so that the obligations of both parties are understood and any legal requirements are completed.

Licence

A lease or sub-lease provides exclusive possession of the leased premises. This means the tenant or sub-tenant can exclude persons (including the landlord) from the leased area subject to a landlord's normal access rights for inspection. If exclusive possession is not required, then one option for a practitioner may be to enter into a licence of required clinic space. A licence allows the owner of land or a tenant as licensor to license a licensee to use land for a particular purpose. This type of arrangement can specify clearly the licensor's and licensee's obligations, but may be less complex and expensive in set-up than a lease. In appropriate situations, this might be sufficient for more casual arrangements. A licence is not binding on a new owner or tenant, and cannot be assigned to another practitioner—unlike a properly created and, if required, registered lease.

Premises requirements for massage and acupuncture

Massage therapy

Specific sanitation and building requirements may apply to premises used by massage therapists or practitioners who use therapeutic massage as part of their practice. In some states, the definition of 'hairdresser' incorporates activities such as massage of the face and scalp. In some cases, massage therapists may be perceived as hairdressers for the purposes of these regulations. The approach taken by the local authorities that administer these regulations is inconsistent.

These requirements may require structural changes, so compliance may be expensive. A search with the local authority is suggested before purchasing a practice that may be subject to these requirements to ascertain whether:

- any licence or qualification is required to carry on business (may be relevant in New South Wales and South Australia), and
- any licence is required for the premises themselves.

The qualifications to obtain a licence to carry on the business (if any) should be ascertained and satisfied. If a licence is required for the premises, a search will reveal whether there is a current licence and any outstanding requisitions or requirements. If a new practice is being established, find out whether a licence is necessary, whether the premises require amendment to comply, and the cost of doing this. Such amendments may require the consent of the landlord.

> **BOX 8.9**
>
> **Practice tip**
>
> If a requirement sought by a local authority appears unreasonable or inconsistent with requirements enforced against colleagues, query it. If you are unsatisfied with the response, you could then seek clarification of the requirement from the council officer or local councillor. Other options include reference to your professional association or ombudsman, and formal legal action.

Skin penetration provisions

Single-use acupuncture needles

Statutory requirements may permit the sterilisation and reuse of needles depending on the jurisdiction; however, a cautious acupuncturist will only use disposable, single-use acupuncture needles. This practice avoids any potential for infections caused by such treatment. Used needles must be disposed of safely in appropriate containers that are not easily accessible to children.

Professional guidelines

The National Health and Medical Research Council's (NHMRC), Australian Guidelines for the Prevention and Control of Infection in Healthcare (2019) (NHMRC Guidelines) do not have the force of law but are an attempt to incorporate most statutory and professional requirements. The NHMRC Guidelines are available at https://www.nhmrc.gov.au/about-us/publications/australian-guidelines-prevention-and-control-infection-healthcare-2019.

Professional guidelines for acupuncturists, Infection Prevention and Control Guidelines for Acupuncture Practice, are also prescribed by the Chinese Medicine Board of Australia. The CMBA guidelines state:

> The National Board has adopted the NHMRC guidelines to inform acupuncturists on infection prevention and control. All registered acupuncturists must comply with:
>
> • the NHMRC Guidelines
> • the National Board guidelines, and
> • relevant state, territory and local government requirements which apply to their place of business.

A copy of these National Board Guidelines, in either printed or electronic form, must be on all premises where acupuncture is practised. Registered acupuncturists in New South Wales, Tasmania, Victoria and the Northern Territory are exempt from the local provisions, while the local regulations still apply in the Australian Capital Territory, Queensland, South Australia and Western Australia. Unregistered complementary medicine practitioners applying techniques involving skin penetration should consider the terms of the NHMRC Guidelines and comply with local regulations.

Local regulations

There are local variations to the standard guidelines, which are dependent upon state law. In most states, there are specific provisions relating to the premises, sterilisation and hygiene applicable to activities involving skin penetration, like acupuncture and dry needling.

NEW SOUTH WALES

The *Public Health Act 2010* (NSW) Part 3 Division 4 and the *Public Health (Skin Penetration) Regulation 2012* (NSW) regulate the practices of those who are not registered as health professionals. The regulation outlines procedures that are to be followed to prevent the transmission of disease. It requires registration of the premises with the relevant local council, and gives power to environmental health officers to inspect the premises. Part 4 of the regulation requires an acupuncturist to:

- notify the local authority of the business address of the premises
- ensure that the premises are clean and hygienic, and
- ensure that any article that penetrates the skin is sterile and is disposed of immediately afterwards or sterilised before reuse.

VICTORIA

Premises used for skin penetration in Victoria must be registered with the local authority. The *Public Health and Wellbeing Act 2008* (Vic) and regulation 24 of the Public Health and Wellbeing Regulations 2019 exempt registered acupuncturists from the requirement to register their premises with the local authority.

Other complementary health practitioners involved in skin penetration are obliged to comply with Part 5, Division 2 of the Public Health and Wellbeing Regulations 2009, relating to the cleanliness of premises, and with the equipment and personal hygiene provisions found in Regulations 29–31. These provisions require a person who uses an article that penetrates the skin to sterilise the article in the manner specified or to dispose of the article immediately.

QUEENSLAND

Under section 148 of the *Public Health Act 2005*, a declared health service includes a service provided to a person to maintain, improve or restore the person's health and involves the performance of an invasive procedure or activity that exposes that person or another to blood or other bodily fluids. Such a service includes those procedures provided at an acupuncture clinic. An acupuncture clinic is deemed to be a healthcare facility under this legislation. Pursuant to section 151, a person involved in the provision of a declared health service must take reasonable precautions to minimise the risk of infection. The owner or operator of such a facility must develop an Infection Control Management Plan (ICMP) before providing the health service. Refer to the following website for details: https://www.health.qld.gov.au/clinical-practice/guidelines-procedures/diseases-infection/infection-prevention/management-plans-guidance/icmp.

The Western Australian Department of Health has published a Skin Penetration Code of Practice, which was developed based on the 1996 National Health and Medical Research Council (NHMRC) Guidelines and contains standards for cleanliness, protection, use of sharps and sterilisation. The code of practice is available at www. health.wa.gov.au.

SOUTH AUSTRALIA

Similarly, the South Australian Health Commission has developed Guidelines on the Safe and Hygienic Practice of Skin Penetration, which provides practice standards. The guidelines are available at www.sahealth.sa.gov.au.

TASMANIA

In Tasmania, sections 104–12 of the *Public Health Act 1997* permit the Director of Public Health to require any person or class of persons to obtain a licence to carry out a public health-risk activity, which is defined to include any activity that may result in the transmission of disease. This licence may include conditions.

NORTHERN TERRITORY

The standards for commercial skin penetration, and hairdressing and beauty and natural therapy are published by Northern Territory Department of Health: Environmental Health. These regulations are exempt for registered health practitioners but apply to unregistered persons involved in procedures including skin penetration.

Occupier liability

As an occupier of premises, a practitioner has potential liability for persons who might injure themselves while on those premises. Liability might arise where a client falls and injures himself or herself on a badly laid carpet, a loose tile or a badly lit set of stairs. Liability could also arise if machinery or equipment causes burns or personal injury, even if the victim is not a client.

Control of premises

Liability for injury is not necessarily based on who owns the land but will often include the person who is in control and occupation of premises. Thus, if a practitioner is leasing or sub-leasing premises, often the tenant rather than the landlord will be liable.

Reasonably foreseeable injury

An occupier's liability is based on what is deemed reasonably foreseeable injury. If it was reasonably foreseeable that a defect in premises might cause injury, the occupier may be liable. A practitioner is required to ensure that premises are in a good state of repair and that activities carried out on those premises are safe. Liability for injury will depend on issues such as:

- whether the defect was obvious and a reasonable adult person would have avoided it, and
- the cost and difficulty for the occupier to remove the danger entirely and to take proper precautions.

The duty of care of an occupier would extend to ensuring that children are not injured on their premises. A balance needs to be found that does not require a too-onerous obligation in relation to protection of children while acknowledging that they do not have the same capacity to understand and avoid danger.

Statutory provisions

The common law of occupier's liability is reflected in statute in a number of states.[6] These statutes indicate that a breach of the duty of care of an occupier is based on matters such as:[7]

- the gravity and likelihood of injury
- the circumstances of entry on to the premises (e.g. whether they were trespassers)
- the nature of the premises
- the knowledge the occupier had or ought to have had that persons would be on the premises
- the age of the person likely to be entering the premises
- the ability of the persons entering the premises to appreciate the danger
- whether the person entering the premises is engaged in an illegal activity (Victoria)
- whether the person entering the premises is intoxicated by alcohol or drugs voluntarily consumed and the level of intoxication (Victoria)
- the burden of eliminating the danger or protecting the person, compared with the risk.

Workplace health and safety

At the federal level and in all states, there is legislation that seeks to secure a safe working environment for people while at work. The Commonwealth *Workplace Health and Safety Act 2011* is intended to provide a national scheme for workplace health

---

BOX 8.10

Practice tip

An occupier can normally assume that a small child will be accompanied by an adult, but should avoid dangers that might be an attraction to children. For this reason, access should be restricted to poisonous substances, hot water, machinery and instruments such as new and used acupuncture needles. A practitioner should take into account that some clients who attend the premises will be sick or in pain, or have a disability.

and safety, which is substantially achieved. In New Zealand, the *Health and Safety at Work Act 2016* applies. Each jurisdiction has a general statute—for instance, in New South Wales the *Workplace Health and Safety Act 2011* and a number of other statutes that deal with specific issues such as agricultural and veterinary chemicals, buildings, mines, dangerous goods and so on. These statutes provide protection for employees by requiring employers/occupiers to abide by the relevant regulations and statutory provisions. This legislation deals with matters such as:

- general safety
- premises safety—walls, floors, ventilation, rest rooms
- plant and equipment—to ensure that these do not injure people while being used
- system of work—to ensure that the way the employees work does not expose them to injury
- materials and substances—steps to avoid poisoning or injury from the substances used, and
- particular issues—such as safe handling to avoid back injury.

There are a large number of standards and specific requirements set for specific tasks. You need to contact your local state workplace health and safety department to ascertain the general and specific requirements for your type of practice. If injury occurs because of a breach of these requirements, the employer/occupier may be liable for that injury.

When considering how to manage health and safety in a small business, consider issues such as the following:

PEOPLE

- Are you employing safe work methods?
- Have the employees been properly trained in their required tasks?
- Have employees been informed of the safety issues in using equipment?
- Do employees require specific licences or permits to use particular equipment or to carry out specific tasks?
- Are clients protected from operational risks, such as exposure to poisons or sharps?
- Have you protected your clients and employees from repair or maintenance contractors?

ACCIDENT REPORTING

Legislation may require reporting of death, serious illness or injury that requires hospitalisation to the relevant government department.

EMERGENCIES

You should have a plan to respond to fire or spillage.

EQUIPMENT

Before purchasing equipment, ensure that it meets any applicable Australian standard and that you understand any potential risks related to its use. Ensure that proper training is given to those who will use the equipment, that the equipment is properly maintained, and that the equipment is regularly inspected to avoid a hazard developing.

MATERIALS

Ensure that handling and storage of materials will not create a hazard for back injuries. This might be achieved, for example, by modifying package size, the use of mechanical aids or storing at waist level to minimise risk.

HAZARDOUS SUBSTANCES

Poisons or other hazardous substances should be labelled and stored correctly to ensure that they do not provide a threat of injury.

Working from home

Many complementary medicine practitioners may wish to avoid the cost and complications of establishing commercial premises and will practise from home. This issue became important in the COVID-19 pandemic when a large percentage of workers worked from home. It is likely the trend of working from home will continue. This approach raises legal issues that should be understood.

Town planning

Each local authority determines what is a permitted use on premises. If a clinic is situated in an area zoned or designated for residential use, using the premises for the practice may be a breach of planning regulations or by-laws. This may result in the local authority imposing a penalty or fine, or requiring the practitioner to cease practice or seek local authority consent. Many practices will proceed without attracting the attention of the local authority. If a complaint is made, an investigation by the local authority may reveal that the use is illegal. Local authority consent may involve an application, advertising of the application and conditions attached to any approval. As local planning regulations vary greatly, it is advisable to contact the local authority to ascertain what might be the relevant regulations that apply to your practice.

BOX 8.11

Practice tip

A complaint to a local authority is most likely to occur where a neighbour complains about traffic or noise from vehicles of clients attending a clinic.

Lease

If the premises are leased under a standard residential lease, check to make sure that the use of premises for business purposes is not a breach of the lease. This may entitle the landlord to terminate the lease. You should consider advising the landlord of your intentions in regard to the use of the property for the practice, though some landlords may not be amenable.

Health requirements

Residential premises used for professional purposes may not comply with local authority and workplace health and safety requirements.

Insurance

Check to ensure that professional indemnity insurance is not voided if procedures are carried out at premises not designed for that purpose. Reference should be made to the relevant insurance policy document. Confirm with your building insurance company that the part of your residential property used for business purposes does not impact on the validity of the policy.

Capital gains tax

By using a residence owned by you partly for business purposes, you may be able to claim a proportion of outgoings (e.g. rates, insurance and repairs) as a business expense. This also means that you may incur a liability for capital gains tax when you sell your home on the proportion of the property used for commercial purposes. You should obtain legal or accounting advice about this issue.

Buying a practice

One option for a practitioner to start or expand a practice is to purchase an existing practice. Whether you are purchasing or selling a business, it is important that you seek professional assistance from an accountant and lawyer. The considerable legal and financial consequences of this transaction require professional advice to avoid unnecessary liability for tax and negative legal consequences.

The contract

The vendor and purchaser will normally enter into a written and binding contract of sale, reflecting the parties' intentions. Prior to contract and in the negotiation stage is the time to ensure that the obligations and undertakings to each other of the vendor and purchaser are understood and reflected in the signed contract. It is difficult to negotiate changes after a contract is signed.

What are you buying?

The first consideration for a purchaser is: What am I buying? Some clarity is required to ascertain whether you are buying goodwill, freehold or leasehold premises, equipment, debts, business name and stock in trade. The answers to these questions determine the steps required to complete the purchase. Both parties need to understand what is or is not included in order to avoid misunderstandings as the transaction proceeds to completion.

The principle 'let the buyer beware' will apply to the transaction. This means that a purchaser should either complete searches on issues of importance prior to entering the contract, or make the contract subject to that issue such as a pest control or building inspection if you are purchasing a freehold property.

To ensure that the business is worth purchasing, ask suppliers and persons in the local community about the reputation of the vendor. To some extent, you are purchasing the vendor's reputation.

Premises

The sale of a business will usually involve a transfer of premises. Considerable goodwill may be attached to this. A clinic well located for the prospective market may attract clients who would not attend a less favourable site. There are two types of premises associated with businesses: freehold and leasehold.

Freehold

If the sale of a business includes a transfer of a freehold interest, the normal conveyancing searches for a purchase of real property are required, including title search, land tax search and local authority search (searches vary from state to state). These searches should be left to a lawyer who is experienced in such matters. The purchase of freehold interest does not transfer any business carried out on the land, so it will require separate documentation.

Leasehold

Most commonly, the practice purchased will be run from leased premises and will involve an assignment of the vendor's lease. Normally, the landlord will need to consent to the assignment of the lease. The purchaser should consider a number of issues in relation to the lease being assigned.

- *Lease term and option*. It would be pointless to purchase a lease that is about to end. Also, some leases need to be registered with the titles office. If such a lease is not registered, the lease and any options to renew may be unenforceable against subsequent landlords.
- *Tenant in default*. If the tenant is in default, the lease could be terminated or the options to renew not exercisable.
- *Landlord's consent*. The contract should be subject to the landlord consenting to the assignment of the lease to the purchaser. The landlord normally cannot refuse consent to the assignment without good reason, such as where there is a concern about the financial viability of the new tenant or because of the proposed use.
- Some leases may prohibit assignments, but this is not common. The lease will usually require an assignee to sign a deed of covenant to observe the terms of the lease. This deed of covenant may contain a personal guarantee of the obligations under the lease by the directors if the assignee is a company.
- *Proposed use*. Confirm that the lease permits the proposed use or that the landlord consents to a change of the use.
- *Town planning*. Confirm that the proposed use is not in breach of local or state planning and environment regulations, planning schemes and legislation. A town planning certificate and other searches with government bodies may be required.
- When a practice has been in existence for a long time at the same premises, the use may not be permitted under a new planning scheme though the original use was

legal when first commenced. This practice may still be permitted as an existing non-conforming use if there has been no cessation or abandonment of the premises or significant change in the scale or type of use. This may require specific inquiries to ascertain the true position. If protection as an existing non-conforming use is not available, the use of the premises for the practice may be prohibited. Reference to local planning legislation and schemes will be necessary and advice from a town planner may be required.

- *Costs of lease.* Obtain details of the rent, outgoings and other costs associated with the lease.
- *Lawyer review.* The purchaser's lawyer should review the terms of the lease to find any unfair or onerous conditions that will affect the purchaser adversely.
- *Goods and services tax.* GST is levied on rent of commercial premises. The lease may provide that the tenant pays this tax.

Contract of sale

The execution of a contract of sale is necessary for the purchase of a business. The important issues that should be considered in preparing this contract are listed below.

Important clauses in contract

- *Parties.* The purchaser and vendor. Advice should be obtained prior to execution by the purchaser to ensure that the business is purchased by the entity that will satisfy legal requirements, provide maximum legal protection and minimise incidence of taxation.
- *Price.* The purchase price may include a component for stock in trade with provision for valuing and payment of stock in trade.
- *Deposit.* Normally a maximum of 10 per cent of the purchase price. Often, a lesser amount may be accepted and lodged with the real estate agent or lawyer for the vendor. The deposit may be forfeited to the vendor if the purchaser defaults under the contract.
- *Date for completion.* Completion is the date when the purchaser pays the vendor the purchase price less the deposit plus stock in trade (if any). This will normally be a period of at least 30 days or longer.
- *Apportionment of purchase price.* For taxation and stamp duty purposes, an apportionment of the sale price between goodwill, plant and equipment, leasehold and stock should be included. This may need to be negotiated between the parties' accountants prior to contract, as it will have income tax consequences for both parties. For the vendor, if the contract provides an apportionment for plant and equipment above their written-down value, this may mean an increased liability for income tax, while for the purchaser there may be advantages in having a higher value for depreciable items to reduce income taxation liability in the future.
- *Warranties.* Warranties are contractually binding statements on matters important to the parties, such as the accuracy of the financial statements.
- Financial statements of the business for the past three years.
- Schedule of plant and equipment to be sold.
- *Assignment of service contracts and warranties.* This relates to service contracts on equipment, such as photocopiers, computers and air-conditioning equipment.

- *Restraint of trade clause.* This limits the vendor's entitlement to practise within a geographic range for a period of time (see page 218).
- *Debts.* Provision as to the debts of the business. Normally, debts will not be sold to the purchaser.
- *Intellectual property.* Transfer of business name and intellectual property such as logos, trademarks and computer software.[8]
- *Finance.* If finance is required, a finance clause should permit a purchaser to terminate the contract and recover the deposit if finance is not forthcoming after reasonable efforts by the purchaser.
- *Special conditions.* Most standard contracts will contain a number of these provisions, but some important special conditions to be contemplated are:

  - obtaining the landlord's consent to assignment of the lease
  - the purchaser being satisfied as to the terms and conditions of the lease
  - obtaining clearances and inspections from relevant bodies such as the local authority or state government health authorities, in regard to matters such as hygiene with required work to be completed at the expense of the vendor; and
  - checking that required local authority planning consents for the practice have been obtained or are in order.

Default

If either party defaults in its obligations under the contract, it may be liable in damages or become subject to legal remedies. If the purchaser fails to pay the balance of the sale price, the vendor may be in a position to terminate the contract, keep the deposit and sue for damages for any loss made on a subsequent sale. The vendor may seek to enforce the contract against the purchaser by seeking a court order requiring the purchaser to complete the contract.

Goodwill

Most sale of business contracts apportion part of the purchase price as goodwill. Goodwill is the likelihood that clients will continue to use the business based on its good name and reputation. Goodwill is a valuable asset, and may be an important element in the value of a business. The likelihood that clients of the vendor will attend the practice will provide revenue and value to the purchaser of that business.

BOX 8.12

Practice tip

The value of goodwill that can be justified on purchasing a business must be considered carefully. The nature of goodwill will depend on the nature of the business. A practitioner may develop close professional relationships with clients, so there must be some doubt about whether clients will use the services of whoever buys the business. Many clients may prefer to follow the former owner of the business, or will go to some other practitioner. If this is likely, then the proportion of the purchase price allocated to goodwill should be small and the purchase price will reflect this.

Financial statements

A contract of sale could contain a warranty that the financial records for the past two to three years attached to the contract are true and correct. This will assist in providing a legal remedy if the records are incorrect or falsified. It is obviously in the interest of the vendor to inflate turnover and profit figures when selling a business. Disappointing trading after purchase could be the result of the change in management, market conditions, the loss of clients who choose to follow the vendor or other reasons. Your accountant should peruse these figures. If possible, a cross-check against appointment books might indicate whether the figures are exaggerated. A perusal of the past two years' records might indicate whether the business is expanding or contracting and at what times of the year it trades best.[9] It will be expensive and difficult to recover damages from a vendor after the sale is completed if financial statements are falsified, so a purchaser should satisfy him or herself in relation to this prior to contract, or make the contract conditional on this point.

Restraint of trade

Any contract to purchase a business should contain a restraint of trade clause. If such a clause is not included, the vendor could start trading nearby immediately after the sale, and this would destroy the goodwill associated with the purchase.

A restraint of trade clause in the context of a sale of business is a covenant by the vendor of the business not to trade in that business for a period of time after completion and usually within a defined radius from the business premises. The clause will be enforceable if it is reasonable as between the parties—that is, it is no wider than necessary to legitimately protect the interests of the parties—and is reasonable in terms of the public interest. For example, a restraint of trade clause for a small acupuncture clinic for twenty years covering a 200-kilometre radius would be unreasonable and unenforceable.

Ensure that the clause is broad enough to limit the vendor being involved in any way in another similar business within the geographical limit specified; otherwise the vendor may be involved in a competing business with, for example, a spouse or family member to the detriment of the goodwill.[10] In New South Wales, refer also to the *Restraints of Trade Act 1976*. This legislation permits a court to determine that an unreasonable restraint of trade is fully or partially unenforceable. Relevant to that consideration is the public interest.

A vendor is obliged not to solicit customers to follow them to another site, though some clients may choose to follow the vendor elsewhere. This will have obvious consequences for the value of the goodwill. If there is concern about this matter, specific reference to what notices can be given to clients can be discussed prior to contract.

Advice period

It may be appropriate to require a vendor to be in attendance for a period after completion to instruct you in the requirements of the business and to introduce you to clients and suppliers.

Debts and liabilities

In most contracts, the debts of the business will not be assigned. The outstanding debts of the business will normally be the responsibility of the vendor. If the purchaser buys the debts of the business, this should be specified in the contract of sale.

If the business has employees, details of wages, holiday pay and long service leave should be made available. Some adjustment to settlement monies may be necessary to cover current liabilities at the date of completion.

Plant, equipment and stock

The contract should cover the assignment of service contracts and warranties for equipment, such as photocopiers, computers and air-conditioning equipment.

PLANT AND EQUIPMENT

The sale of a business will often involve a transfer of some plant and equipment such as massage tables, chairs and desks. A search should be made under the name of the vendor to ascertain whether there is any security over these assets and whether the vendor owns these goods. Warranties from the vendor about the ownership of these assets should be obtained. If plant and equipment is subject to security, they should be paid out.

STOCK

If the parties intend to transfer stock in trade, such as herbs and vitamins, provide for a stocktake and valuation on the completion date. Normally, the costs of that exercise are borne equally. Take care to purchase only stock that is saleable.

Fees and taxes

Goods and services tax: sale of business

In some circumstances, GST will be levied on the sale price of a business even if the parties have not included the tax in the purchase price. The imposition of GST will not occur where it is established that:

* the sale of the business was for money or money's worth
* the purchaser is a registered person under the GST system or someone required to be registered, and
* it was a sale of a going concern where the parties have agreed in writing to that effect.

The sale of a going concern occurs when the vendor supplies all things that are necessary for the continued operation of the business and the vendor continues the business until sold. A sale involving isolated assets or not including goodwill would not qualify for exemption from GST. These requirements suggest that the sale of a practice after the death of a practitioner may not qualify for the exemption, as the business is not a going concern.

Stamp duty

The purchaser will pay stamp duty on the transfer of the business based on the sale price, including stock in trade.

Goods and services tax

A practitioner will be obliged to recover GST on professional services unless exempt, as discussed on page 221. All practitioners will be subject to payment of GST on purchase of non-exempt equipment, stock and supplies. A practitioner needs to understand whether they are exempt, the limits of that exemption and how to recover GST paid on purchases for the practice.

BOX 8.13

Action plan

Taxation

- Obtain an Australian Business Number (ABN) under Goods and Services Tax (GST) provisions.
- Register the business for GST (if appropriate).
- Set up accounting systems for the business and trading structure.

What is GST?

The GST is levied at a standard rate of 10 per cent in Australia on all goods and services, except for those foods and some services specifically exempted. GST is paid by the end-user and will be part of the displayed price. Businesses will pay GST on their purchases of goods or services, charge GST on each sale made, remit the GST payable to the Tax Office and claim GST credits for those purchases. GST must be accounted for every time a practitioner makes a 'taxable supply' of goods or services, unless the transaction is exempt. Every time a practitioner who is registered for GST incurs an expense on a purchase that includes GST, the practitioner will be entitled to a credit for the GST part of the cost (called an 'input tax credit'). A simple transaction by a naturopath registered for GST on non-exempt substances might look like this:

> *Herbal mixture manufacturer* sells product for $5.50 including 50 cents for GST (GST to ATO assuming no input tax credit).
> *Naturopath* buys mixture for $5.50 including GST.
> *Consumer* buys mixture for $11 including $1 GST (naturopath remits $1.00 less 50 cents input tax credit to ATO).
> Total $1.00 to ATO.
> Total $1.00 paid by consumer.

Persons, partnerships and companies, including professionals such as complementary medicine practitioners who carry on business, are required to register for GST if their turnover in a twelve-month period is in excess of $75,000. Hobbies or recreational activities are excluded from this requirement where there is no expectation of profit or gain. If the business has a turnover less than the threshold, it is optional to register. Practitioners may choose to register even if the turnover threshold will not be reached to obtain credits for GST paid on purchases associated with the practice. A practitioner unregistered for GST does not need to recover GST on sales or send any GST to the Tax Office. Practitioners should find out from their accountant whether they must or should register for GST and their obligations under the law.

Obtaining an Australian Business Number

Even if a practitioner opts not to register for GST, it may be necessary to obtain an ABN. Without an ABN, when you provide goods or services to another business, they will retain the maximum rate of income tax on the money payable to you. You will have to wait for a refund of this amount when lodging your tax return.

If purchasing goods, herbs and equipment that are subject to GST, a practitioner, if registered, can obtain a GST credit on the purchases. The practitioner must have an invoice for the purchase in the required format, showing the GST that has been levied.

Exemptions

In Australia, section 38.10 of the *A New Tax System (Goods and Services Tax) Act 1999* confirms that the supply of health services for chiropractic, osteopathy, acupuncture, naturopathy or herbal medicine (including traditional Chinese herbal medicine) is GST-free if:

* the supplier is a recognised professional in relation to the supply of services of that kind, and
* the supply would generally be accepted, in the profession associated with supplying services of that kind, as being necessary for the appropriate treatment of the recipient of the supply.

A 'recognised professional' is a professional who has permission, approval or registered status under state or territory legislation, or is a member of a professional association with uniform national registration requirements in relation to the supply of services of that kind. A number of major professional associations have been acknowledged by the Australian Taxation Office as providing appropriate uniform national registration requirements so as to deem their members 'recognised professionals'. Practitioners should check whether membership of an association that they intend to join or have joined provides them with status as a 'recognised professional'.

The supply of goods associated with the supply of the exempt professional services may also be exempt from GST for chiropractic, osteopathy and acupuncture if the supply is made at the premises at which the service is supplied (the clinic). This would presumably include the supply of acupuncture needles, vitamins and supplements. For herbal medicine, including TCM and naturopathy, the supply of goods such as medicine or herbs is GST-free if the goods are supplied in the course of supplying the services and if they are supplied and used or consumed at the premises.

The GST-free status does not apply to services supplied by massage therapists and homoeopaths. Note that the exemption applies to the service, not the practitioner.

This would presumably mean that the supply of massage services by an acupuncturist would not be exempt, and the supply of homoeopathic remedy advice by a naturopath would also not be exempt.

Instalment Activity Statements and Business Activity Statements

If you are registered for GST you may be required to lodge a Business Activity Statement (BAS) monthly, every quarter or annually, depending on your circumstances. The BAS will determine the amount of GST and Pay-as-You-Go (PAYG) income tax that you may be required to pay. If you are not registered for GST and you earn income through your practice, you will be obliged to lodge an Instalment Activity Statement (IAS) every quarter to determine the level of PAYG income tax that is payable. Depending on your level of income, you may be permitted to lodge an annual IAS or simply rely on your annual income tax return. These provisions are complex and a full treatment is not possible here. You should seek advice from an accountant about your obligations.

New Zealand provisions regarding GST

New Zealand also has a GST which applies to a broader range of goods and services than that applying in Australia. GST in New Zealand is added to taxable goods and services at a rate of 15 per cent. In New Zealand, taxable goods and services include all types of personal and real property and services except money. Taxable goods and services don't include goods and services supplied by a business not registered for GST and exempt supplies for letting or renting a dwelling house for use as a private home, interest, donated goods and services sold by a non-profit body and certain financial services.

A person must register for GST if they carry out a taxable activity and their turnover is over $60,000 for the past twelve months or is expected to go over $60,000 for the next twelve months. In addition, persons who have a turnover of less than $60,000 but have included GST in their prices should register for GST. Turnover is the total value of taxable supplies excluding GST, and will normally be the total value of sales and income. A person with a turnover of less than $60,000 may choose to register for GST.

GST is charged on taxable activities, being activities carried out continuously or regularly by a business, professional, association or club, and involves the supply of goods or services for a consideration but not necessarily for a profit. As in Australia, parties registered for GST in New Zealand are obliged to lodge a GST return and pay the required GST by the due date for the relevant taxable period.

The New Zealand Internal Revenue website provides good advice about the requirements for the New Zealand GST regime at www.ird.govt.nz/gst.

Employees

Liability for employees

An employer will often be legally responsible for acts of an employee based on the concept of vicarious liability, even if the employer is not at fault in any way. For example, a chiropractor would be liable for the negligent acts of a masseur employed to perform massage prior to manipulation. If a receptionist were to reveal confidential information about a client's medical history, the employer would probably be liable for any legal consequences of that breach.

BOX 8.14

Action plan

Employees

- Prepare employment contracts (if appropriate).
- Put in place systems for wages, long-service leave and superannuation requirements.
- Make sure locums are appropriately qualified and trained, and hold a provider number for health insurance refunds (if relevant).
- Make sure employees have registered status if required.
- Provide for workers' compensation and superannuation payments.
- Research appropriate wage levels for employees.

Independent contractors

Vicarious liability does not extend to the acts of a party who is not an employee but an independent contractor. It is sometimes difficult to differentiate between an independent contractor and an employee, but the determination can have an important bearing on the liability of the employer. An independent contractor carries out work as a principal, and his or her negligence will normally not create liability for the employer.

A familiar example of an independent contractor is an electrician who installs a new electrical connection or a plumber who fixes a leaking tap. These persons are employed to perform a specific task, and they act with limited or no supervision from the householder.

Traditionally, the distinction between independent contractors and employees was based on the control test. If the worker was told what he or she was to do and how to do it, then he or her was probably an employee. An independent contractor was employed to complete a particular task but was not subject to order or control as to how the work was to be done. This test is now somewhat out of date. Today, the appropriate test involves a complex assessment of a number of issues such as:

- Was the person part of the employer's business—suggesting employee?
- How did the parties consider their relationship (e.g. did the employer withhold tax—suggesting employee?)
- Was the person subject to the orders of the employer as to where, when and how the task was approached—suggesting employee?
- Did the employer have a power of dismissal—suggesting employee?
- An employee does not bear financial risk while an independent contractor bears that risk.
- Generally an employee will have standard or set hours while an independent contractor will determine how many hours to complete a project.
- The parties determine to create an employee/employer relationship or the opposite—suggesting an employee.

- Did the employee supply his or her own tools or equipment? This may suggest an independent contractor.
- Could the person select their own subordinates or delegate? This suggests an independent contractor.
- Was the party in business on his/her own account? This suggests an independent contractor.

The Fair Work Ombudsman provides an overview of the criteria to determine if the person is an independent contractor or employee. https://www.fairwork.gov.au/find-help-for/independent-contractors

Locums

Clearly, there is no degree of control over the activities of the locum, as the primary practitioner is not normally present. The contract of employment might clearly indicate whether the locum was an independent contractor or employee. The locum will probably be an independent contractor where he or she:

- maintains separate professional indemnity insurance
- is paid fees rather than weekly wages from which amounts for taxation and superannuation are not deducted, and
- is carrying on a business in his or her own right.

A practitioner would be safer to assume that he or she is vicariously liable for the acts of the locum as an employee. Most professional indemnity insurance policies make specific provision for indemnity for this liability. Note the limits to this cover that relate to employment of a locum beyond 60 aggregate or 30 consecutive days during the period of insurance. Any agreement with a locum should confirm their duty not to poach clients at the end of their contract period.

BOX 8.15

Practice tip

A locum should:
- be properly qualified, otherwise the indemnity available in any insurance policy may be voided
- have a medical benefits fund provider number so clients can obtain refunds
- be aligned to the clinical and business approach of the practice, and
- be a member of an appropriate professional association.

Acting outside the limits of employment

Once it is established that the relationship is one of employer and employee, the employer will be vicariously liable for the acts of the employee, i.e. the employer is liable for negligence by a an employee within the course of their employment. The courts are generally reticent to interpret an act as outside the course of employment so as to avoid liability for an employer.

It is difficult to determine when an act is within the course of employment. The question is whether the employee has done something that is unrelated to the task for which they are employed. For example, a massage therapist employed to massage may step outside the scope of her employment if she prescribes herbs.

An employer's vicarious liability may not affect the potential personal liability of an employee for their negligence. A plaintiff will often prefer to seek recovery from the employer as they may have access to professional indemnity insurance or greater personal assets. In New South Wales, South Australia and the Northern Territory, solvent or insured employers are obliged to protect employees from claims unless they involve 'serious and wilful conduct' by the employee or, in New South Wales, if it did not occur in the course of, and did not arise out of, the employment of the employee.[11] Similarly, section 66 of the *Insurance Contracts Act 1984* (Cth) provides that an insurance company cannot seek to recover from the employee the pay-out they may have made under a general insurance policy unless the employee's acts were wilful or serious misconduct.

Professional indemnity insurance

Every complementary medicine practitioner should maintain professional indemnity insurance for the benefit of both the practitioner and client. This insurance can provide peace of mind and protection for the practitioner not available to a self-insured practitioner. Protection may be vital, even where a practitioner has not been negligent. For example, without the protection of professional indemnity insurance, the practitioner may be subject to legal costs for dealing with frivolous or unfounded claims. This section will discuss general principles, but every insurance policy is different so practitioners need to make reference to the particular wording of their policy and obtain specific legal advice.

Purpose of professional indemnity insurance

In return for payment of the premium, the insurance company should:

* defend claims made against the insured practitioner (normally, the insurance company will undertake the conduct of the matter for the practitioner with his/ her cooperation)
* provide the services of a lawyer to oversee any litigation that may ensue (some policies allow the practitioner to nominate a lawyer with the insurance company's consent), and
* satisfy a claim up to the maximum limit specified by the policy, for a negotiated settlement or a court determination.[12]

The insured practitioner is obliged to:

* refrain from specified acts or activities that may prejudice the insurance company, such as making admissions of liability
* report incidents or potential claims promptly, and
* cooperate with the insurance company in defending any claim made.

Most professional associations require a practitioner to maintain professional indemnity insurance. Some professional associations arrange access to a common master policy for all members. In the absence of a policy, any liability arising out of the practice must be satisfied from the assets of the practitioner.[13]

Maintenance of a professional indemnity insurance policy is essential for all practitioners, although the policies:

*   may appear difficult to understand or decipher
*   involve payment of premiums (for complementary medicine practitioners, the premiums are normally relatively inexpensive)
*   may involve a minor loss of freedom of practice, and
*   require the completion of forms and documents.

What does the policy cover?

*   *Liability in the course of practice.* The policy should cover liability for a breach of the practitioner's duty of care in the course of their practice, causing bodily or mental injury or death. Coverage does not extend to acts of the insured in their private capacity. For example, a chiropractor who gives investment advice to clients will not be covered for any liability for this advice.[14] The policy will normally provide coverage to the policy's monetary limit for a claim within the terms of the policy, plus the costs and expenses of the defence of the claim.
*   *Nuisance or crank claims.* Some practitioners think that, because they provide a high standard of service using safe and gentle techniques, professional indemnity insurance is not necessary or worthwhile. But an insurance policy can protect against a nuisance or crank claim of no substance. Without professional indemnity insurance coverage, the considerable cost of defending such a claim would be borne by the practitioner.
*   *Partners and employees.* The policy will normally cover the person specified as the insured; members of a partnership, company or corporation specified as insured; employees; and locums. In some cases, employees and locums may be obliged to undertake to be bound by the insurance policy before being covered.
*   *Competition and Consumer Act 2010 (Australian Consumer Law)* and *Fair Trading Acts.* Commonly, an extension of the policy includes claims made against the practitioner pertaining to the *Competition and Consumer Act 2010* (Cth) or *Fair Trading Acts* involving misleading and deceptive conduct.
*   *Coronial and disciplinary proceedings.* The policy relevant to chiropractors and osteopaths extends to the costs associated with disciplinary proceedings or a coronial inquiry against the practitioner arising out of the practitioner's practice to a stated maximum liability for costs.
*   *Students.* Many policies have an extension for the teaching of students.
*   *Liability for libel or slander.* Many policies provide cover for libel and slander in some circumstances.

What doesn't the policy cover?

*   *Monetary limit.* Amounts payable outside the maximum limits of the stated coverage are not covered. Seek advice from your professional association as to the level

of coverage. Some policies provide for an 'excess' that the practitioner is obliged to satisfy where a claim is made against the policy. Most policies have automatic reinstatement provisions that may allow protection for amounts in excess of the limit of indemnity for subsequent claims.

- *Activities outside professional practice.* Activities outside the scope of the professional practice specified in the policy will not be covered. This is an issue of some importance. Practitioners should clearly understand the professional scope of their professional indemnity insurance policy. Some insurance policies cover virtually any complementary medicine modality or therapy likely to be applied. Other policies have a much more limited scope—for example, a policy in relation to a herbalist will not necessarily cover services such as therapeutic massage. A claim made in relation to an activity outside the scope of the policy may be refused. Although the courts tend to take a broad approach to interpreting the scope of a professional practice clause, the burden is on the insured to show that the activity came within the scope of the policy.[15] If the policy relates to a registered profession, the relevant statutory scope of practice may influence the assessment of the activities covered by the policy.
- *Dishonesty of insured.* A professional indemnity policy cannot indemnify against the dishonesty of the insured, as this would be against public policy. Normally such policies do, as an extension, allow coverage in relation to the dishonest act of an employee, including loss of money or negotiable instruments.
- *Contracts.* The cover may not include liability under contract where there would otherwise have been no liability. This could occur where a practitioner has contracted to produce a specific result and has been unsuccessful, though not negligent, and would not otherwise have been liable in any way.
- *When intoxicated.* Any services provided while the practitioner is under the influence of drugs or intoxicants are not covered.

What if the practitioner wants to proceed to trial and the insurance company wants to settle?

Based on a practitioner's assessment of the claim and a feeling of moral outrage, he or she may prefer to proceed to trial. The insurance company may agree that the claim has little validity but prefers an early settlement, bearing in mind the inherent risks and expense of litigation.

Most policies allow a practitioner to proceed to trial with the consent of the insurance company on the basis that they will limit their liability to what would have been a settlement sum plus costs to that date. Any further costs or damages awarded would be the responsibility of the practitioner. A practitioner should be very cautious before proceeding to trial against the advice of the insurance company.

Different types of policy

Occurrence and 'claims made' policies

There are two types of professional indemnity insurance policy that should be understood, as the differences can create problems in coverage.

OCCURRENCE COVERAGE

An 'occurrence coverage' policy provides protection for an incident during the period of the insurance policy, even if a claim arising from that incident is made at some future date. Thus, if a policy is in place in 2021 and an incident occurs in that year, there is coverage for a claim made in subsequent years resulting from that incident. This type of insurance is normally more expensive as the insurance company cannot quantify its potential liability for a number of years.

CLAIMS MADE

A 'claims made' policy is more common. This type of policy provides protection for a claim made (i.e. a summons, statement of claim or other court document or a written or verbal demand for compensation) during the term of the policy. If an incident occurs in 2021 and no claim is made in that year, the insurance company may not be liable under a policy in existence in 2021. If a claim arising from the 2021 incident is made in 2022 and no policy is then in existence, there may be no coverage. If the insured has renewed the policy, the claim made in 2022 for the incident in 2021 may be covered under that renewed policy. As the insurance company is aware of its liability for claims in each year, this type of policy is usually provided at a lower premium. Some policies extend protection for claims made after the year of coverage arising out of circumstances occurring in the year of coverage, if the insurance company is notified of those circumstances before the end of the period of cover. For that reason, you should advise the insurer (whether the same insurer or subsequent insurer) promptly of that potential claim to assist the enforceability of coverage under any subsequent policy.

It is important for a practitioner to understand the basic parameters of their cover and, if necessary, to obtain legal advice. Practitioners need to be aware of the possibility of gaps in coverage in the following situations. Legal advice or advice from an insurance broker may be required to deal with the following gaps so that appropriate coverage can be maintained:

- *When a practitioner switches from a 'claims made' to an occurrence policy.* The 'claims made' policy does not apply to the claims made after the end of the prior policy, and the occurrence policy will not provide coverage except in relation to events during the new policy period.
- *When a practitioner retires with a 'claims made' policy.* In this case, he or she may not be covered for claims made in subsequent years for incidents occurring in the years prior to retirement.
- *When practitioners enter a partnership at one time or over a period of time.* Many policies provide coverage for retiring and new partners, subject to conditions.

These problems suggest that frequent switching between insurance companies should be avoided if possible.

Continuous cover

Most policies have a continuous cover clause, which provides an incentive not to change insurance companies. This clause applies to a claim made in regard to an incident prior to the commencement of the policy, where the same insurer was the insurer when the insured became aware of the circumstances subsequently giving rise to the claim, and the insurer has been the insurer uninterrupted since that date. This clause allows that the claim will be met subject to the policy in existence when the claim is made.

Obligations

All insurance policies, including professional indemnity, are contracts of utmost good faith. It is essential that the insured answers all questions honestly in any proposal form completed before the policy is taken out. The insured is obliged to reveal all known facts material to the risk being undertaken under the policy.

The purpose of this obligation is to reveal to the insurer the risk it is undertaking under the policy before entering that obligation. These facts may only be known by the insured. For example, whether questioned by the insurer or not, the insured should reveal any history of claims or any possible claim pending.

Educating insurance company and lawyers

A practitioner may need to educate the insurance company and the lawyers about their modality and the differences in approach from standard medical procedures. An ignorance of some of the basic precepts of the profession may prejudice efforts to successfully settle, negotiate and litigate the claim.

Public liability, premises and contents insurance

Many policies contain an extension for public liability to cover injuries suffered while on the practice premises and for product liability—that is, coverage for bodily injury or damage to property caused by goods sold or supplied in connection with the practice. Some policies will incorporate building, contents and practice insurance coverage.

What to do when a claim is made

Despite their best efforts, a practitioner may become involved in an incident that has the potential to create liability in negligence. It may be a case of:

* a clearly negligent act by the practitioner
* an overly sensitive and worried client
* a practitioner clearly not being at fault, or
* the practitioner's position being doubtful or unclear.

It is appropriate to discuss the initial steps that should be taken by the practitioner, as this may impact on the result of ensuing litigation. The major points for practitioners to remember are:

* *Don't panic.* For every circumstance that might create a liability for negligence, only a small percentage will eventuate in a claim actually being made. If a practitioner panics, and makes inappropriate comments or statements, this may increase the chances of a claim successfully being made.

- *Contact your professional indemnity insurance company immediately.* It is in the interest of the insurance company to assist the practitioner in dealing with the matter satisfactorily from an early date.
- *Show sympathy to the client.* This will give the client the opportunity to vent their feelings and for the practitioner to gather details of the alleged injury. Contact with the client requires some care, as statements could be made that will suggest an admission of guilt. Even if the practitioner thinks they have made a mistake, it is ultimately for a court to determine this if in the rare case the matter proceeds to trial. In relation to the use of apologies, refer to the discussion on page 115 above. In some jurisdictions, an apology may be inadmissible in court, though it is still important not to admit fault in discussions with clients. There are differing views as to whether contact should be made with a client in the early stages after an incident. Most clients do not want to sue their practitioner. For some clients, sympathetic and caring concern at this stage will reduce any likelihood of further action, while for others such attention will have little bearing on their approach.
- *Advise other partners and professional and administrative staff.* Informing them of the need to be sympathetic and helpful without providing any admission of guilt is advisable. Avoid admissions of guilt even to staff members, as they may be called as witnesses. If the event was caused by some breakdown in office procedure, take steps to avoid this happening again. If the event was caused by a staff member, this person may need counselling to deal with anguish that may result, and appropriate training if this is indicated.
- *Don't attempt to 'doctor' client records after the event.* There may be a temptation to adjust the client file to present yourself in a better light. This temptation should be resisted on a number of bases:

  - Such an act is morally wrong and a serious breach of professional ethics.
  - If presented as a true and honest record in court proceedings, it may constitute the criminal offence of perjury.
  - Tampering is difficult to perform without being found out.
  - Technology today (e.g. determining the age and type of paper used) can be used to detect alterations and later insertions. The discovery that records have been tampered with would have a devastating effect on the credibility of a practitioner in litigation or in negotiating a settlement.
  - Losing a file may also create an impression that the loss was intended. Such a loss means that the matter must be resolved using the oral testimony of the practitioner and other witnesses. This will occur in circumstances where the loss of the file may suggest, at best, that a practitioner was unprofessional and, at worst, that they were involved in a designed and dishonest attempt to hide unfavourable evidence.

Resources

One of the best sites in Australia is the Queensland government site at business.qld. gov.au, which provides a 'Step by Step Guide' to starting a business. This is directly relevant to Queensland practices but may also provide an indication of relevant issues for other states.

Notes

1 *Business Names Register Act 2011* (Cth) section 16.
2 *Corporate Affairs Commission v Bradley* [1973] 1 NSWLR 382 at 389.
3 https://www.servicesaustralia.gov.au/chronic-disease-gp-management-plans-and-team-care-arrangements#a5.
4 https://ablis.business.gov.au/ (accessed 6 November 2021).
5 www.ato.gov.au/business/starting-your-own-business/business-or-hobby.
6 *Wrongs Act 1958* (Vic), Part II A; *Civil Liability Act 1936* (SA), Part 4; *Occupiers Liability Act 1985* (WA) s 5.
7 Vic, s 14B; SA, s 20; WA, s 5.
8 L. Ball, 'Buying a Practice' (1998) 4 *Journal of the Australian Traditional Medicine Society* 2, 56 at 57.
9 Ibid.
10 Ibid.
11 *Employees Liability Act 1991* (NSW), ss 3, 5; *Civil Liability Act 1936* (SA), s 59; *Law Reform (Miscellaneous Provisions) Act* (NT), s 22A.
12 L. Campbell, C. Ladenheim, R. Sherman & L. Sportelli, *Risk Management in Chiropractic: Developing Risk Management Strategies*, Health Services, Fincastle, VA, 1990, p. 45.
13 Ibid.
14 D. Derrington & R.S. Ashton, *The Law of Liability Insurance*, Butterworths, Sydney, 1990, p. 566.
15 Ibid.

Index

Printed in the United States
by Baker & Taylor Publisher Services